Johannes Zschocke
Georg F. Hoffmann

Vademecum
Metabolicum

3rd Edition

Vademecum Metabolicum

**Diagnosis and Treatment
of Inborn Errors of Metabolism**

3rd, revised Edition

**Johannes Zschocke, Innsbruck, Austria
Georg F. Hoffmann, Heidelberg, Germany**

Foreword by
William L. Nyhan, San Diego, USA

Contributors:
Alberto B. Burlina, Padova, Italy
Roberto Giugliani, Porto Alegre, Brazil
Martin Lindner, Heidelberg, Germany
Yoichi Matsubara, Sendai, Japan
Ertan Mayatepek, Düsseldorf, Germany
Shamima Rahman, London, UK
Wolfgang Sperl, Salzburg, Austria
Jerry Vockley, Pittsburgh, USA
Kurt Widhalm, Vienna, Austria
Ed Wraith, Manchester, UK

With 29 figures and 40 tables

Johannes Zschocke, Dr. med. habil., PhD
Professor and Chair of Human Genetics
Medical University Innsbruck
Schöpfstraße 41, 6020 Innsbruck
Austria

Georg F. Hoffmann, Dr. med. habil.
Professor and Chair of Paediatrics
Ruprecht-Karls-University
Im Neuenheimer Feld 430, 69120 Heidelberg
Germany

This edition corresponds to the fourth German and Italian editions.

Bibliographic information published by the Deutsche Nationalbibliothek. The Deutsche Nationalbibliothek lists this publication in the Deutsche Nationalbibliografie; detailed bibliographic data is available in the Internet at <http://dnb.d-nb.de>.

Important note:
Medicine is an ever-changing science, so the contents of this publication, especially recommendations concerning diagnostic and therapeutic procedures, can only give an account of the knowledge at the time of publication. While utmost care has been taken to ensure that all specifications regarding drug selection and dosage and treatment options are accurate, readers are urged to review the product information sheet and any relevant material supplied by the manufacturer, and, in case of doubt, to consult a specialist. The publisher will appreciate – also in the public's interest – to be informed of possible inconsistencies. The ultimate responsibility for any diagnostic or therapeutic application lies with the reader.

© 1999, 2004, 2011 by Milupa Metabolics GmbH & Co. KG, 61381 Friedrichsdorf, Germany
www.milupa-metabolics.info
Printed in Germany
First unaltered reprint 2014 of the 3rd edition 2011

Composing: Bernd Burkart; www.form-und-produktion.de
Printing and binding: CPI – Ebner & Spiegel, Ulm
Printed on paper bleached without chlorine or acid.

ISBN 978-3-7945-2816-5

Foreword

It is my pleasure to write the Foreword for the third edition of the *Vademecum Metabolicum*. This very useful book has now been translated into many languages including German, English, French, Italian, Hungarian, Portugese and Japanese. It has continued to grow in scope, as has the field of inborn errors of metabolism. At the same time, it has remained true to its original objective of providing a systematic approach to the diagnosis of metabolic disease. The book is still small enough to fit in a pocket, and has become a favourite of physicians in training in Paediatrics and Genetics. Revisions have brought the book up to date, impressively so in the disorders of glycosylation, neurotransmission, and vitamin metabolism. Extensive tabular presentation leads the reader logically to the diagnostic possibilities. Optimal therapy, including dosages, makes for a well rounded approach to the various diagnosis and management of genetic diseases of metabolism.

University of California, San Diego, USA **William L. Nyhan, MD, PhD**

Preface

Inborn errors of metabolism, which cumulatively affect approximately one in every 500 newborns, represent a special challenge in general and paediatric practice. They frequently present with acute, life-threatening crises that require immediate specific intervention. The development and prognosis of the affected child may depend on rapid and effective treatment, but the large number of genetic defects in various biochemical pathways makes it difficult to be familiar with all diagnostic strategies and specific therapies. With this in mind, the *Vademecum Metabolicum* aims to provide practical guidance to the clinician.

This 3rd English edition has been completely revised and expanded. As in previous editions, the first section on the diagnosis and management of metabolic disorders includes clinical situations that may be caused by a metabolic disorder. Practical guidelines are discussed in detail and should reflect standard practice in many countries. The second section on individual metabolic pathways and their disorders has been completely revised and includes a considerable number of recently identified disorders. As in the previous editions, special emphasis has been placed on clinical features that are relevant to a whole group of diseases, useful diagnostic procedures (basic and special diagnostic tests) as well as details on emergency intervention and long-term treatment. The pathobiochemistry is described in more detail when it is relevant to the understanding of clinical symptoms and diagnostic tests. The sequence of the entries is either according to metabolic pathways or nomenclature.

The genetic basis of most disorders in the Vademecum Metabolicum has now been clarified, and the causative genes have been included when known. Throughout the text we have removed references to molecular studies as part of the diagnostic strategy since mutation analyses are now a standard option for confirmation of most metabolic disorders. Inheritance of the disorders is autosomal recessive unless specified otherwise.

We are grateful to Marinus Duran, Amsterdam, James V. Leonard, London, Verena Peters, Heidelberg, Jan A. M. Smeitink, Nijmegen, Udo Wendel, Düsseldorf, and Nicole Wolf, Amsterdam, who contributed to previous editions of this book. Again we are indebted to Dr. Beate Szczerbak, Milupa, Friedrichsdorf, for her unwavering, continuous support. The friendly and professional help of Claudia Ganter, Birgit Heyny and Klaus Jansch at Schattauer Publishing, Stuttgart, is gratefully acknowledged.

Innsbruck and Heidelberg, August 2011   **Johannes Zschocke**
Georg F. Hoffmann

Table of contents

Abbreviations

AA	amino acids
AFP	α-fetoprotein
ALT	alanine aminotransferase
AST	aspartate aminotransferase
BH$_4$	tetrahydrobiopterin
Bioch.	biochemistry
BW	body weight
Cbl	cobalamin
CDG	congenital disorders of glycosylation
CK	creatine kinase
CoA	coenzyme A
Compl.(s)	complication(s)
Confirm.	confirmatory studies
CPT	carnitine palmitoyltransferase
CSF	cerebrospinal fluid
DBS	dried blood spot
DD	differential diagnosis
DH	dehydrogenase
Diagn.	diagnosis
FA	fatty acids
FFA	free fatty acids
Fru	fructose
GABA	γ-aminobutyric acid
GAG	glycosaminoglycans
Gal	galactose
GALT	galactose-1-phosphate uridyltransferase
GC	gas chromatography
Glc	glucose
HMG	3-hydroxy-3-methylglutarate
HPLC	high performance liquid chromatography
IEM	inborn error of metabolism
i.m.	intramuscular
Indic.	indication
i.v.	intravenous
IVA	isovaleric aciduria
Lab.	laboratory
Manif.	manifestation
MCAD	medium-chain acyl-CoA DH
Metab.	key metabolites
MMA	methylmalonic aciduria
MPS	mucopolysaccharide(-osis)
MRI	magnetic resonance imaging
MRS	magnetic resonance spectroscopy
MS	mass spectroscopy
mth(s)	month(s)
n	normal

NH$_3$	ammonia
NMR	nuclear magnetic resonance
OA	organic acids
OH-	hydroxy-
OTC	ornithine transcarbamylase
P	phosphate
PA	propionic aciduria
PALP	pyridoxal phosphate
PC	pyruvate carboxylase
PDH	pyruvate dehydrogenase
PKU	phenylketonuria
Progn.	prognosis
SCAD	short-chain acyl-CoA DH
SCHAD	short-chain hydroxyacyl-CoA dehydrogenase
SIDS	sudden infant death syndrome
Tx	transplantation
Var.	variant
VLCAD	(very)-long-chain acyl-CoA dehydrogenase
wk(s)	week(s)
yr(s)	year(s)

Amino acids

Ala	alanine
Arg	arginine
Asa	argininosuccinic acid
Asn	asparagine
Asp	aspartate
Cit	citrulline
Cys	cysteine
Gln	glutamine
Glu	glutamate
Gly	glycine
Hcy	homocysteine
His	histidine
Ile	isoleucine
Leu	leucine
Lys	lysine
Met	methionine
Orn	ornithine
Phe	phenylalanine
Pro	proline
Ser	serine
Tau	taurine
Thr	threonine
Trp	tryptophan
Tyr	tyrosine
Val	valine

Diagnosis and management of metabolic disorders

Essential basic laboratory tests

The following basic laboratory tests should be performed in every child with an acute illness in whom a metabolic disorder is a possibility:

Blood glucose
Hypoglycaemia is a presenting feature of several disorders particularly of carbohydrate and energy metabolism. Appropriate blood and urine samples should be obtained in the acute phase to make the correct diagnosis. *For details see page 5.*

Ammonia
Ammonia is highly neurotoxic and hyperammonaemia carries a high but in principle avoidable mortality and morbidity. Urgent analysis of the plasma ammonia concentration is mandatory in all acutely ill neonates and all patients with undiagnosed encephalopathy. Facilities to determine ammonia at any time of the day should be available in all hospitals. Hyperammonaemia due to a primary urea cycle disorder is among the most urgent emergencies in metabolic paediatrics and will be missed if ammonia is not measured. *For details see page 7.*

Acid-base status
Many metabolic disorders cause alterations in the acid-base status, both acidosis and alkalosis. Blood gas measurements need to be available at any time in every hospital. *For details see page 10.*

Lactate
Elevated lactate is an important sequel of hypoxia and compromised energy metabolism and may be the cause of metabolic acidosis. A primary metabolic disorder should be considered if there is no convincing secondary cause such as shock, asphyxia or cardiac disease or in particular a difficult venepuncture. *For details see page 11.*

Urinary ketones (test strip)
Ketonuria due to the ketone bodies 3-hydroxybutyrate and acetoacetate is normal during fasting but is pathological in the fed state and in the neonate where it may indicate a disorder of intermediary metabolism. Absence of ketones during fasting is suggestive of a fatty acid oxidation disorder. Ketone levels measured by non-specific tests (e.g. test strips) may be high due to the presence of interfering compounds. *See also page 11.*

Other laboratory tests
Organ dysfunction caused by metabolic disorders may be recognised in routine investigations such as blood counts, liver function tests, coagulation studies or creatine kinase levels. Uric acid is elevated in several disorders with increased cellular turnover or decreased urinary clearance. *See also page 28.*

Specific triggers of metabolic decompensation

Triggers	Groups of disorders
Vomiting, fasting, infection, fever, vaccination, surgery, accident/injury	Disorders of protein, energy or carbohydrate metabolism or hormone homoeostasis
High protein intake and/or protein catabolism	Disorders of protein metabolism: aminoacidopathies, organic acidurias, urea cycle defects, hyperinsulinism-hyperammonaemia syndrome
Fruit, table sugar (sucrose), liquid medicines	Fructose intolerance
Lactose, milk products	Galactosaemia
High fat intake	Lipoprotein lipase deficiency, glycerol intolerance, fatty acid oxidation disorders
Drugs	Porphyrias, Glc-6-P-dehydrogenase deficiency
Extensive exercise	Disorders of fatty acid oxidation, glycolysis, muscle glycogenolysis, purine and pyrimidine metabolism, respiratory chain

General clinical situations

The metabolic emergency

In the neonate, the early clinical features of acute metabolic decompensation are almost always non-specific; they include "unwell", lethargy, feeding problems, vomiting, abnormal breathing, hypotonia and seizures. Disorders of glucose, protein and fat breakdown (intermediary metabolism) in the neonatal period typically have an *asymptomatic interval*, with clinical manifestations from the second day of life onwards ("intoxication type"), although hyperammonaemia in particular may present as early as day 1. The baby's general condition will usually deteriorate rapidly despite normal or non-specific findings in routine investigations (laboratory signs of infection, lumbar puncture, chest X-ray, cranial ultrasound) and antibiotic therapy. The *family history* may reveal siblings who died with similar clinical manifestations ("sepsis", "SIDS") or unexplained disorders in other family members (progressive neurological disease, maternal PKU, multiple miscarriages, HELLP syndrome, etc.). Consanguinity increases the risk of a recessive disorder.

Metabolic disorders **after the neonatal period** may present with recurrent vomiting and lethargy progressing to coma without focal neurological signs or typical patterns of organ dysfunction. Initial management may follow similar principles as in neonates. Care must be taken to identify the conditions that triggered metabolic decompensation such as vomiting and fever or changes in the diet.

A metabolic disorder should be considered, along with other diagnoses (e.g. infection, CNS pathology) ...
... in all neonates with unexplained, overwhelming or progressive disease particularly after normal pregnancy and birth;
... in all children with acute deterioration of the general condition and/or reduced consciousness, particularly when preceded by vomiting, fever or fasting;
... in all children with symptoms and signs of acidosis or hypoglycaemia.

Appropriate diagnostic and therapeutic measures must be initiated as soon as possible to avoid long-term damage.

Post-mortem investigations: see *page 25*

Phase 1: Basic metabolic emergency investigations and first line management
Stop intake of potentially toxic compounds (protein, fat, galactose, fructose)

Insert i.v. line and take blood samples for urgent analysis of:
• Electrolytes, *glucose*, CRP, CK, ALT, AST, creatinine, urea, uric acid, *acid-base status*, coagulation studies
• Ammonia, lactate
• Store plasma sample for amino acids, acylcarnitines, etc.
• Store filter paper card ("Guthrie" card for newborn screening) with dried blood spots for acylcarnitines (amino acids, possibly DNA studies)
• Store the rest of the other samples for possible additional tests (inform laboratory)

Obtain urine sample:
- Check colour and odour
- Perform standard test strip analyses (e.g. ketone bodies, glucose, protein; pH > 5 during acidosis → DD renal tubular acidosis)
- Store urine sample from the acute phase for organic acids or additional metabolic tests

If lumbar puncture is performed:
- Store CSF (freeze immediately)

Start with **10% glucose infusion, 150 ml/kg/day** (10 mg/kg/min, ~60 kcal/kg/day), with appropriate electrolytes.

   Glucose supply in this infusion is at the rate of normal hepatic glucose production and is usually sufficient for disorders of reduced fasting tolerance such as glycogen storage disorders or MCAD deficiency. It may not be sufficient in disorders that are exacerbated by catabolism, e.g. organic acidurias or urea cycle defects. It may be potentially dangerous in mitochondrial disorders (specifically pyruvate dehydrogenase deficiency) as a high glucose supply may enhance lactic acidosis. The benefits of the high-glucose infusion outweigh the risks but lactate and acid-base status should be checked regularly.

Order additional investigations as indicated, e.g. ECG, echocardiogram, cranial imaging. **Results of emergency investigations should be available within 30(–60) min**. At that stage, decide on specialist investigations and additional therapeutic measures.

Phase 2: Treatment and investigations according to the initial findings

If the emergency investigations show ...
... hypoglycaemia: see *page 5*
... hyperammonaemia: see *page 7*
... metabolic acidosis: see *page 10*
... elevated lactate: see *page 12*
... severe liver disease: see *page 19*

If results are inconclusive but metabolic disease remains a possibility:
- Continue glucose infusion
- Review the history and clinical signs. Phone regional metabolic centre for advice.
- After discussion, send samples for specialist metabolic investigations (results relevant to the diagnosis of treatable metabolic disorders should be available within 24 [at most 48] hrs):
  – Dried blood spots for acylcarnitines and amino acids (urgent analysis)
  – Plasma sample for amino acids and acylcarnitines
  – Urine sample for simple metabolic tests and organic acids
- Monitor electrolytes, glucose, lactate, acid-base status (keep sodium well above 135 mmol/l to avoid cerebral oedema)

Hypoglycaemia

Definition
Blood glucose <2.6 mmol/l (45 mg/dl) at all ages

> Glucose concentration:
> 1 mmol/l = 18 mg/dl
> 10 mg/dl = 0.55 mmol/l

Consider
- *In the neonate*: evidence of non-metabolic causes?
- *History*: time since last meal (hypoglycaemia postprandial, after fasting), drugs, erratic?
- *Examination*: hepatomegaly, liver failure or cirrhosis, small genitals, hyperpigmentation, short stature?
- *Glucose requirements*: >10 mg/kg/min indicates (persistent or transient) hyperinsulinism (*page 88*) unless there are marked losses elsewhere (e.g. urine)
- *Rule out* (in the neonate): septicaemia, severe systemic illness, small for gestational age, maternal diabetes

Laboratory investigations during symptomatic hypoglycaemia
Adequate laboratory tests must be carried out *during symptomatic hypoglycaemia* to identify the underlying cause, or else many diagnoses may be missed.

Essential
- **Free fatty acids + 3-hydroxybutyrate** (serum or plasma); ketones (test strip). A marked elevation of *free fatty acids* indicates active lipolysis and that the hypoglycaemia is associated with a fasting reaction. In this situation, "normal" (low) values of *plasma ketones* (3-hydroxybutyrate is sufficient) are strongly suggestive of a disorder of fatty acid oxidation or ketogenesis. Normal values: see *page 167*.
- **Acylcarnitines** (dried blood spots or plasma). This test is diagnostic of most (but not all) fatty acid oxidation disorders and various organic acidurias.
- **Hormones** (serum). *Insulin* (normal: insulin completely suppressed when glucose <2.6 mmol/l [45 mg/dl]), *cortisol* (normal >270 nmol/l).
- **Lactate** (blood, NaF tube). Elevations may indicate liver damage or impaired glycogenolysis/gluconeogenesis but may also be found after a seizure or difficult blood sampling (see *page 12*).
- **One spare tube** (serum or plasma) for anything from below or forgotten or lost
- **Organic acids** (urine) → various metabolic disorders that may cause hypoglycaemia

Others
- Blood gases, blood count, CRP, electrolytes, phosphate, liver/renal function tests, CK, uric acid, triglycerides, carnitine status, growth hormone
- Ammonia (EDTA blood) → e.g. liver damage or glutamate dehydrogenase deficient hyperinsulinism
- Amino acids (plasma)
- Consider toxicological investigations (incl. C-peptide)

Differential diagnosis

Hypoglycaemia in premature children is frequently caused by problems of adaptation and may not require extensive laboratory tests. The most frequent causes of persistent neonatal hypoglycaemia are hormonal disturbances, e.g. hyperinsulinism or hypopituitarism. Hypoglycaemia of hyperinsulinism is accompanied by low concentrations of free fatty acids and ketone bodies due to *inhibition of lipolysis*. *Regulatory disturbances* (e.g. ketotic hypoglycaemia, glycogen storage disease type III, hypopituitarism after the first year of life) result in hypoglycaemia with particularly strong ketosis. *Defects of fatty acid utilisation* (*carnitine shuttle, fatty acid oxidation, ketogenesis*) are characterised by hypoglycaemia, high levels of free fatty acids and low ketones during lipid catabolism. *Gluconeogenesis defects* (e.g. glycogen storage disease type I) show marked hypoglycaemia with lactic acidosis; ketone levels may be low or elevated.

As always: There are exceptions to every rule or simplification.

Ketones "normal" (low) or insufficiently elevated		**Free fatty acids relatively low**: hyperinsulinism, ↓ counter-regulatory hormones
		Free fatty acids greatly elevated: disorders of fatty acid oxidation and ketogenesis
Ketones elevated		"Ketotic hypoglycaemia", organic acidurias, ↓ counter-regulatory hormones (after the first year), glycogen storage disease types III and 0, ketolysis defects
Lactate elevated (>2 mmol/l)	Without hepatomegaly	Organic acidurias, ketolysis defects, respiratory chain defects, long-chain fatty acid oxidation disorders (especially LCHAD)
	Isolated hepatomegaly	Glycogen storage diseases, gluconeogenesis defects
Liver disease		Fructose intolerance, respiratory chain defects, long-chain fatty acid oxidation disorders, tyrosinaemia type I

Treatment
- Glucose i.v. 7–10 mg/kg/min (glucose 10%: 110–150 ml/kg/day), keep blood sugar ≥ 5.5 mmol/l (100 mg/dl).
  If glucose bolus is needed: Do not give more than 200 mg/kg (glucose 20%: 1 ml/kg).
- Await results of specialist investigations and treat accordingly
- High glucose requirement > 10 mg/kg/min or incompletely suppressed insulin at times of hypoglyaecemia is abnormal and suggests hyperinsulinism (see *page 82*)
- For disorders of fatty acid oxidation and ketogenesis see *page 91*

Hyperammonaemia

NH_3 concentration: μmol/l = μg/dl × 0.59

NH_3 values:	*Neonates*:	Healthy	<110 μmol/l
		Sick	up to 180 μmol/l
		Suspect metabolic disease	>200 μmol/l
	After the neonatal period:	50–80 μmol/l	
		Suspect metabolic disease	>100 μmol/l

Blood sample: Uncuffed venous (or arterial) sample, keep on ice, analyse immediately.

Caution: NH_3 concentration in tissue is 10× higher than in blood. False elevations of ammonia are common.

> It is essential to measure ammonia early in every sick child in whom a metabolic disease may be the underlying diagnosis. Hyperammonaemia may be missed otherwise and the child may be deprived of efficient treatment. If it is not possible to obtain the "perfect sample": Measure ammonia anyway and repeat under better circumstances if ammonia is high.

Causes

- *Urea cycle disorders (page 57)*: Most common cause of severe hyperammonaemia, presenting with progressive or chronic relapsing encephalopathy. May initially be associated with respiratory alkalosis (central effect of hyperammonaemia) but metabolic alkalosis or acidosis may occur. Short time-span from first symptoms to irreversible brain damage – rapid and efficient management is of utmost importance!
- *Organic acidurias and long-chain fatty acid oxidation defects* (e.g. propionic aciduria; *page 62*) – approx. 30% of severe neonatal hyperammonaemias: Blocked urea synthesis due to deficiency of acetyl-CoA (required for N-acetylglutamate synthesis) and inhibition of NAGS by organic acids. Usually associated with (lactic) acidosis at an early stage (*note*: Sometimes alkalosis due to vomiting or hyperammonaemia). The ammonia concentration does not allow a diagnostic distinction between urea cycle defects and organic acidurias. In general glutamine is not increased in organic acidurias or fatty acid oxidation disorders.
- *Hyperinsulinism-hyperammonaemia syndrome* (HIHA; glutamate dehydrogenase deficiency): NH_3 values rarely above 200 μmol/l
- *Severe liver failure* (*note*: Elevated transaminases or reduced PTT may also be found in urea cycle defects)
- *Transient hyperammonaemia* due to open ductus venosus, particularly in neonates with respiratory distress syndrome – plasma-Gln/NH_3 ratio <1.6 μmol/μmol
- *Increased muscle activity* during assisted ventilation, respiratory distress syndrome or shortly after generalised seizure – NH_3 values rarely above 180 μmol/l

Emergency investigations and differential diagnosis

A metabolic disorder should be *strongly suspected in all term babies with NH_3 > 200 μmol/l*. As treatment differs for different causes of hyperammonaemia, it is important to reach the exact diagnosis as soon as possible. The results of all laboratory investigations must be obtained within a few hours, if necessary at night. **Contact the metabolic specialists (emergency services) by phone, send samples by courier (taxi)!**

Investigations
- Basic investigations (*page 3*)
- Amino acids in plasma and urine
- Organic acids and orotic acid in urine
- Acylcarnitines in dried blood spots

Differential diagnosis

Plasma citrulline	Other features	Diagnosis
Low (usually)	↑↑ Orotic acid	Ornithine transcarbamylase deficiency
	Specific acylcarnitines and organic acids	Organic aciduria, e.g. propionic or methylmalonic aciduria
	↓–n Orotic acid	Carbamylphosphate synthase deficiency N-acetylglutamate synthase deficiency Ornithine aminotransferase deficiency (newborns)
$> 30 \ \mu M$	↑ Orotic acid	Lysinuric protein intolerance
$> 50 \ \mu M$	↓–n Orotic acid, ↑ lactate	Pyruvate carboxylase deficiency (neonatal)
$100–300 \ \mu M$	↑ Argininosuccinate	Argininosuccinic acidaemia
$> 1,000 \ \mu M$	↑ Orotic acid	Citrullinaemia

Emergency management

Organise all treatment options as soon as hyperammonaemia is confirmed. Extracorporeal detoxification must be promptly initiated with NH_3 >500 μM. Even conservative therapy requires frequent monitoring of ammonia and plasma amino acids, and the patient should usually be *transferred to the nearest paediatric metabolic centre*. Insert central venous catheter and arterial line.

Principles
- Stop protein intake, reduce catabolism
- Remove ammonia (drugs, extracorporeal detoxification)
- Replenish urea cycle intermediates with arginine or citrulline; support mitochondrial metabolism with carnitine in organic acidurias
- Support urinary ammonia excretion by generous fluid intake; consider forced diuresis

First infusion
- Glucose 10 mg/kg/min (10% solution: 12 ml/kg/2 hrs) with appropriate electrolytes

Over 2 hrs
- L-Arginine hydrochloride 360 mg/kg (= 2 mmol/kg = 2 ml/kg of 1 M solution)
- Na-benzoate 250 mg/kg
- Na-phenylacetate 250 mg/kg i.v. (or oral Na-phenylbutyrate 250 mg/kg)
- L-Carnitine 100 mg/kg (less when fatty acid oxidation disorder may be present)
- Consider Ondansetron (Zofran®) 0.15 mg/kg i.v. bolus in the non-comatose child (infusion can lead to nausea and vomiting)

L-Arginine HCl, Na-benzoate (and carnitine) should be diluted in glucose 5% 35 ml/kg BW and administered as a bypass to the regular infusion.

Check glucose, add insulin if necessary; check ammonia after 2 hrs.

Note: Na-benzoate and -phenylacetate (precursor *Na-phenylbutyrate* available only for oral administration in most countries) provide alternative pathways of nitrogen excretion by conjugation with glycine and glutamine, respectively. There has been some debate whether these substances should be used for detoxification of ammonia before the diagnosis is known because there is the *theoretical risk of intramitochondrial CoA depletion in organic acidurias.* However, in many metabolic centres these drugs are regularly used for the detoxificion of ammonia in organic acidurias (especially propionic aciduria), without apparent adverse effects. Na-benzoate and phenylbutyrate/-acetate are *toxic* in high plasma concentrations (above 2 mmol/l and 4 mmol/l, respectively). Measuring plasma levels of Na-benzoate is recommended in the neonatal period, particularly in jaundiced infants, but this analysis is not available in most centres. The risk of toxicity is considered to be low with maintenance doses of 250 mg/kg/day but may be relevant with higher doses. *Check for high serum-Na$^+$ and low K$^+$* particularly during treatment with both Na-benzoate and -phenylbutyrate (250 mg/kg Na-benzoate or -phenylbutyrate contain 1.74 mmol or 1.35 mmol sodium, respectively).

Extracorporeal detoxification

Start urgently if NH_3 >500 µmol/l (>850 mg/dl). Use haemodiafiltration if available, otherwise haemofiltration or haemodialysis. Peritoneal dialysis is not efficient. Exchange transfusion increases the protein and ammonia load and should not be used.

Consider oral *carbamyl glutamate* 100–200 mg/kg as a starting dose followed by 100–200 mg/kg/day in 3–4 doses ($T_{1/2}$ = 5–6 hrs) in patients with biochemical findings suggestive of CPS I or NAGS deficiency (acute hyperammonaemia, normal orotic acid, absence of specific other metabolites; see *page 60*) or in every patient when results of special biochemical investigations are not available within hours.

Maintenance treatment of hyperammonaemia

Maintenance infusion (over 24 hrs)

* *Arginine hydrochloride* (180–)360 mg/kg (adjust according to plasma Arg levels: aim for 80–150 µmol/l; stop once argininaemia or lysinuric protein intolerance has been diagnosed)
* *Na-benzoate* 250 mg/kg (up to 500 mg/kg in confirmed urea cycle disorders, provided that plasma levels can be monitored); Na-phenylacetate/-phenylbutyrate 250 mg/kg when i.v. preparation available; otherwise oral Na-phenylbutyrate 250–500 mg/kg/day in 3 doses when possible.
* *Carnitine* 100 mg/kg/day (not required once urea cycle defect is confirmed)
* *Glucose* 10–20(–30) g/kg, add insulin 0.1–1 IU/kg/hr if blood sugar >150 mg/dl or glucosuria
* *Intralipid* 0.5–1 g/kg after exclusion of long-chain fatty acid oxidation disorder (up to 3 g/kg – monitor triglycerides)
* Adequate amounts of fluids and electrolytes
* If necessary: *antiemetic therapy* with Ondansetron (Zofran® 0.15–0.5 mg/kg)

Treatment after diagnosis: urea cycle defects see *page 58*, organic acidurias see *page 61*.

The prognosis in terms of neurological complications and psychomotor development is good if coma duration was <36 hrs before start of specific therapy, or more specifically, if the concentration of NH_3 (µmol/l) multiplied with the duration of coma (days) has remained <2,400 µmol/l.

Metabolic acidosis and ketosis

Normal values:	pH	7.37–7.43
	PaO_2	70–100 mmHg (9.3–13.3 kPa)
	$PaCO_2$	27–40 mmHg (3.6–5.3 kPa)
	HCO_3^- (arterial)	21–28 mmol/l
	Anion gap = $[Na^+] - [Cl^- + HCO_3^-]$	7–16 mmol/l

Metabolic acidosis is characterised by decreased pH, HCO_3^- and $PaCO_2$.

Differential diagnosis

Acidosis due to	Typical findings
Renal loss of bicarbonate	Normal anion gap, increased Cl^-, urinary pH > 5 (with acidosis); *renal Fanconi syndrome*: additional signs of renal tubular dysfunction (↑ urinary glucose, reducing substances, phosphate, amino acids)
Intestinal loss of bicarbonate	Diarrhoea; normal anion gap, increased Cl^-; urinary pH may be elevated due to hypokalaemia and secondary increase of urinary ammonium
Organic acids (e.g. lactate, ketones)	Increased anion gap

Renal causes of metabolic acidosis

Presenting feature of
- Various forms of primary renal tubular acidosis (= RTA, various modes of inheritance)
- Fanconi-Bickel disease (glycogenosis type XI due to a deficiency of glucose transporter Glut2; causes RTA, aminoaciduria, phosphaturia, glucosuria, fasting hypoglycaemia; see *page 85*)
- Lowe syndrome (oculocerebrorenal syndrome: RTA, cataracts, glaucoma, hypotonia)
- Osteopetrosis (RTA, typical bone changes)
- Cystinosis (see *page 141*)

Accompanying feature of
- Tyrosinaemia type I (see *page 68*)
- Hereditary fructose intolerance (see *page 81*)
- Glycogen storage disease type I (see *page 83*)
- Mitochondrial disorders (see *page 96*)
- Methylmalonic aciduria (chronic renal damage; see *page 62*)

Metabolic acidosis caused by accumulation of organic anions
Increased anion gap > 16 mmol/l

Acquired causes
• Severe infections, septicaemia
• Advanced catabolic state
• Tissue hypoxia
• Dehydration
• Intoxication

Investigations: Determine causative acid(s)
• Blood lactate
• Blood ketones (3-hydroxybutyrate)
• Urinary organic acids
• Plasma amino acids
• Carnitine status (free and total)
• Acylcarnitines (dried blood spots)

Differential diagnosis (primary metabolic disorders)

Ketones	Lactate	Other organic acids	Blood glucose	NH_3	Suggestive diagnosis
+–++	(n–)++	++	Variable	n–↑	Organic acidurias (MMA, PA, IVA)
+++	n	++	Variable	n–↑	Oxothiolase deficiency
+++	n–↑	++	High	Low	Diabetes mellitus
n–++	+++	Variable	Variable	n–↑	Respiratory chain disorders, pyruvate dehydrogenase deficiency
n–++	++	Variable	Low	n	Disorders of gluconeogenesis or glycogen storage
Low	n–++	+	Low	n–↑	Fatty acid oxidation defects

Ketosis
Ketosis is a physiological response to fasting, catabolic state or ketogenic diet. In some children ketosis is associated with nausea and vomiting; "ketonaemic" vomiting of infants with normal blood sugar is rarely caused by a primary metabolic disorder. Permanent ketosis may in rare cases indicate a ketolysis defect. Ketosis in addition to other metabolic abnormalities is frequently found in disorders that affect mitochondrial metabolism (particularly organic acidurias but also e.g. respiratory chain disorders). The differential diagnosis includes diabetes mellitus. *Ketonuria in the neonate is often indicative of a primary metabolic disorder.*
Ketosis with fasting hypoglycaemia due to benign regulatory disturbances is found as a normal variant in infants and small children but may also indicate adrenal insufficiency or glycogen storage diseases (GSD) type 0. Postprandial ketosis and lactic acidosis in association with fasting hypoglycaemia and hepatomegaly may indicate GSD III or other GSD types (see also *page 83*).

Elevated lactate

Lactate concentration: mmol/l = mg/dl × 0.11

Normal values: *Blood* <2.1 mmol/l (<19 mg/dl)
                     CSF <1.8 mmol/l (<16 mg/dl)
Blood sample: Uncuffed vein (scalp, i.v. line) or artery, relaxed child
                     Na-fluoride sample tube

Pyruvate analysis is not usually indicated. Measurement may be considered when lactate is elevated to determine the lactate/pyruvate ratio (redox state, normal <20). This requires perchloric acid extraction (see also *page 37*).
Alanine (plasma amino acids) reflects the concentration of pyruvate (and indirectly lactate) but is not affected by cuffing. Normal <450 µmol/l, alanine/lysine ratio <3.

Differential diagnosis

It can be difficult to distinguish primary and secondary lactic acidaemia. CSF lactate should be determined routinely when a lumbar puncture is performed in patients with neurological disease.

Secondary causes
- Most common: the use of a tourniquet or difficulty in drawing the blood
- Muscular activity, assisted ventilation, seizures (lactate up to 4–6 mmol/l)
- Severe systemic disease: central and peripheral hypoxia or ischaemia, shock, cardiac failure, cardiomyopathy, liver or renal failure, septicaemia, diabetes mellitus, etc.
- Any severe metabolic disease
- Renal tubular syndrome, hyperchloraemia, urinary tract infection (lactic aciduria)
- Drugs (biguanides); intoxication (e.g. ethanol)
- Consider thiamine deficiency (see also *page 161*)

Metabolic causes
- Disorders of the respiratory chain or Krebs cycle
- Pyruvate dehydrogenase (PDH) or pyruvate carboxylase deficiency
- Long-chain fatty acid oxidation disorders
- Organic acidurias, disorders of biotin metabolism
- Glycogen storage diseases, gluconeogenesis disorders

Laboratory investigations
- *Acylcarnitine analysis* will reliably detect most disorders of fatty acid metabolism.
- *Severe ketosis* is indicative of a primary metabolic disorder (inhibiton of the Krebs cycle). It is not usually found in fatty acid oxidation disorders.
- *Postprandial elevation* of lactate (>20%) or ketone bodies (paradoxical ketonaemia) may indicate PDH deficiency or respiratory chain defects, respectively.↑ Lactate after glucose challenge is found also in glycogen storage disease types 0, III, VI.
- *Postprandial decline* of lactate concentrations and fasting hypoglycaemia may indicate glycogen storage disease type I or gluconeogenesis defects.

Treatment

Treat according to the primary diagnosis. For details on the diagnosis and treatment of primary lactic acidosis or mitochondrial disorders see *page 96*.

Intellectual disability

Many metabolic disorders cause variable, chronic brain damage and intellectual disability. This may be progressive (continuous or exacerbated by acute illness), sometimes involving loss of previously acquired skills and typically affects all areas of development to a variable extent. The parents may report severe behavioural problems such as hyperactivity, irritability, aggressiveness or sleep disturbances. Careful neurological examination may reveal objective anomalies, e.g. of muscle tone. Involvement of other organs should be sought by clinical examination. Additional investigations such as abdominal ultrasound scan or skeletal X-rays should be guided by clinical findings. Clinical genetic evaluation and possibly genome-wide array analyses are generally useful in children with significant intellectual disability. MRI, extended metabolic studies, EEG and neurophysiological tests are only indicated in severely affected children.

Laboratory tests in isolated intellectual disability without dysmorphic features
- Basic laboratory tests (*page 1*)
- Check thyroid function
- Creatine metabolites (urine; → creatine transporter deficiency; *page 111*)
- Genetic analyses, e.g. DNA array, fra(X) syndrome
- Consider lysosomal disorders (*page 129*)

Additional laboratory tests in intellectual disability with neurological abnormalities
- Consider additional genetic analyses, e.g. Rett syndrome, Angelman syndrome (check lists)
- Urine: simple tests, organic acids, glycosaminoglycans, oligosaccharides, sialic acid
- Plasma/serum: quantitative amino acids
- Biotinidase activity, if not included in newborn screening (dried blood spots)
- Consider purines and pyrimidines (urine), glycosylation disorders (CDG; *page 146*)
- Consider thiamine deficiency (see also *page 161*)

Additional laboratory tests in intellectual disability with dysmorphic features
- Sterols, peroxisomal studies (very long-chain fatty acids, phytanic acids, plasmalogens)
- Transferrin isoelectric focusing for glycosylation studies (CDG; *page 146*)
- Other genetic analyses, e.g. screening for subtelomeric deletions

Intellectual disability and ...
   ... progressive loss of skills or organomegaly: consider lysosomal disorders (*page 129*)
   ... multi-system disorder: consider mitochondrial disorders (*page 96*), peroxisomal disorders (page 143), glycosylation disorders (CDG; *page 146*)
   ... liver disease (see *page 19*)
   ... progressive myopia, dislocated eye lenses: measure total homocysteine (*page 33*)
   ... cardiomyopathy (see *page 17*)
   ... abnormal hair: consider Menkes disease (*page 162*)
   ... seizures (see *page 14*)
   ... macrocephaly: check urinary organic acids (glutaric aciduria type I, Canavan disease, etc.), lysosomal storage diseases. MRI is recommended as hydrocephalus must be ruled out. One of the recently identified leukodystrophies, megalencephalic leukodystrophy with subcortical cysts (MLC) can only be diagnosed by MRI.

Metabolic (epileptic) encephalopathy

Epileptic seizures occur frequently in many metabolic disorders but are particularly common with disorders of the cerebral grey matter. All children with epilepsy and additional symptoms such as failure to thrive, intellectual disability, dysmorphic features or neurological abnormalities should be examined by brain MRI and receive a metabolic work-up incl. CSF analyses.

Indications for neurometabolic (CSF) studies
- Neonatal progressive encephalopathy
- Neonatal or infantile epilepsy that is refractory to treatment, infantile myoclonic epilepsy
- Extrapyramidal movement disorders, e.g. parkinsonism-dystonia, dyskinesia and hypokinesia, progressive dystonia, chorea, hypotonia, ataxia, rigidity, muscular hypertonia (extremities)
- Ptosis, miosis, oculogyric crises
- Disturbances of autonomic regulation, e.g. hypersalivation, disturbed intestinal motility, disturbances of temperature regulation

Investigations in blood and urine
- Basic laboratory tests (*page 1*), incl. repeated ammonia, lactate
- Standard clinical chemistry, incl. Ca, Mg, Cu, uric acid, coeruloplasmin, alkaline phosphatase
- Plasma amino acids incl. homocysteine (centrifuge and freeze)
- Simple urine tests (incl. bedside sulphite test for sulphite oxidase deficiency; *page 71*)
- Urinary organic acids (4-hydroxybutyrate, vanillyllactic acid, N-acetylaspartic acid)
- Urinary purines and pyrimidines, creatine metabolites
- Peroxisomal studies (very long chain fatty acids)
- Serum glycosylation studies (CDG; *page 146*)
- Biotinidase activity (dried blood spots)
- Pipecolic acid and aminoadipic acid semialdehyde (urine, plasma, CSF, freeze samples immediately!)
- Prolactin in serum (secretion is dopamine-dependent)
- Whole blood serotonin (altered in pterin defects, monoamine oxidase and aromatic L-amino acid decarboxylase deficiencies)

Investigations in CSF
(A detailed guide to CSF investigations for neurometabolic disorders has been published by Hoffmann et al. *Neuropediatrics* 1998; 29: 59–71)
- Routine investigations incl. cytology, immunology, protein chemistry
  - CSF glucose <2.7 mmol/l or CSF/plasma ratio ≤0.45 in glucose transport protein deficiency
- Lactate; if elevated consider pyruvate
- Amino acids (specific sensitive analysis required, concurrent CSF + plasma samples)
  - Glycine CSF/plasma ratio (normal <0.04, neonate <0.08; elevated in non-ketotic hyperglycinaemia; *page 74*)
  - Serine CSF/plasma ratio <0.2 in serine synthesis defects (*page 74*)
  - Alanine and threonine (mitochondrial disorders)
- Biogenic amines and metabolites in CSF: neurotransmitter disorders (see *page 151*)
- Pterins (special sample tube), possibly also in plasma and urine
- 5-Methyltetrahydrofolate <5 nmol/l: cerebral folate transport (FOLR1) deficiency and other disorders of folate metabolism (*page 157*)
- Pipecolic acid and aminoadipic acid semialdehyde; antiquitin deficiency (*page 160*)

CSF – sample preparation and shipment

In contrast to inborn errors in catabolic pathways, neurotransmitter defects are reflected by the interplay of biosynthesis, degradation and receptor status. Even borderline abnormalities can be diagnostic and their recognition requires a strictly standardised sampling protocol and adequate age-related reference values. The concentrations of several metabolites change with the respective CSF fraction (rostro-caudal gradient). It is therefore essential to exactly label the CSF samples (fractions) that are sent to the laboratory. Freeze CSF sample immediately at the bedside (no additives – dry ice), store at –70 °C. If blood-stained: centrifuge before freezing (inform laboratory).

Age < 1 yr: collect 0.5 ml fractions, use fractions 2–5 for metabolic investigations.

Age > 1 yr: collect 1 ml fractions, use fractions 3–6 for metabolic investigations.

Ship on dry ice.

Special metabolic investigations
- Phenylalanine loading test (see *page 47*)
- Serotonin in EDTA whole blood
- Free GABA in CSF

Other investigations
- Magnetic resonance spectroscopy of the brain allows the regional semi-quantification of various metabolites incl. creatine, lactate and various neurotransmitters. It was central to the discovery of disorders of creatine metabolism.
- NMR spectroscopy of CSF and other body fluids is a powerful method to identify known and unknown key metabolites and has led to the identification of several novel disorders, e.g. of polyol metabolism.

Differential diagnosis of epileptic encephalopathy – consider
- Neuronal ceroid lipofuscinoses (*page 140*)
- Other lysosomal disorders (*page 129*)
- Peroxisomal disorders (*page 143*)
- Mitochondrial disorders (*page 96*)
- Choreoacanthocytosis (*page 29*)

Treatment of epileptic encephalopathy – try
- Pyridoxine 100(–500) mg i.v., and/or folinic acid 3 mg/kg i.v.: vit. B_6-responsive seizures, antiquitin deficiency (*page 160*)
- Pyridoxal phosphate 30 mg/kg oral: pyridoxal phosphate-responsive seizures (*page 160*)

The floppy infant

Muscular hypotonia is a common symptom in metabolic disorders in which it is usually associated with other symptoms such as lethargy or coma, seizures, neurological abnormalities or dysfunction of other organ systems. Laboratory investigations may identify typical metabolic derangements. Isolated muscular hypotonia is more frequently observed in primary neuromuscular disorders or the Prader-Willi syndrome.

Investigations
- Basic laboratory tests (*page 1*), electrolytes, CK
- Urine: simple tests, organic acids, oligosaccharides
- Plasma: quantitative amino acids
- Serum: carnitine (free and total), peroxisomal studies (*page 36*)
- Dried blood spots: acylcarnitines, biotinidase activity

Consider
- Mitochondrial disorders (*page 96*), disorders of (long-chain) fatty acid oxidation and the carnitine cycle (*page 91*)
- Pompe disease (*page 84*), peroxisomal disorders (*page 143*); CDG (*page 146*)
- Causes of epileptic encephalopathy (*page 14*)

Exercise intolerance

Exercise induced pain, muscle cramps and destruction of muscle fibres may be caused by insufficient energy supply of muscle cells.

Differential diagnosis
- Muscle glycogenoses (*page 85*)
- Disorders of fatty acid oxidation, e.g. carnitine palmitoyltransferase II (*page 92*)
- Mitochondrial disorders (*page 96*)
- Disorders of purine nucleotide cycle: myoadenylate deaminase deficiency (*page 114*)

Enquire
- When does pain start?
  - Disorders of glyco(geno)lysis: symptoms typically occur at start of intense exercise; may improve after short rest ("second wind" phenomenon)
  - Disorders of fatty acid oxidation: symptoms typically occur during longer exercise and in recovery phase
  - Disorders of respiratory chain: ability to exercise continuously compromised
- Discolouration of urine after exercise (myoglobinuria)?
- Other problems, e.g. haemolytic anaemia (disorders of glycolysis), Reye-like episodes (disorders of fatty acid oxidation)?

Investigations
- "Muscle enzymes" incl. CK, LDH + isoforms, aldolase, ALT/SGOT, AST/SGPT, urea creatinine, thyroid hormones; myoglobin (urine): elevated during/after episodes
- Acylcarnitines (dried blood spots)
- Molecular genetic analyses

Cardiomyopathy

Cardiomyopathy is an important manifestation of several metabolic disorders. It is often dilated hypertrophic and may be associated with severe arrhythmia. Skeletal myopathy is usually also present but may be subtle. It is important to search for additional signs of systemic disease incl. hepatic or neurological dysfunction, storage disease or metabolic derangement.

Endocardial fibroelastosis: Thickening and stiffening of the endocardium in various conditions incl. metabolic disease, viral myocarditis, or "idiopathic".

Differential diagnosis

Disorder/groups	Additional features (not mandatory)	Age (yrs)	Page
Pompe disease (infantile)	Very floppy, typical ECG	0–1	84
Fatty acid oxidation	Encephalopathy, fasting hypoglycaemia, lactic acidosis, liver dysfunction	0–2	91
Mitochondrial	Lactic acidosis; heart block	Any age	80
Barth syndrome	3-Methylglutaconic acidurias; neutropenia	0–2	63
MPS I, II and VI	Features of "storage disorder"	Any age	130

Accompanying feature in:

Disorder/groups	Additional features (not required)	Page
Organic acidurias (e.g. propionic)	Metabolic acidosis, ketosis	61
Haemochromatosis	Liver disease	163
Congenital disorders of glycosylation	Multi-system disease; pericardial effusion	146
Glycogen storage disorders types III + IV	Hepatomegaly, hypoglycaemia	83
Lysosomal disorders	Cardiac involvement may be valvular and may be mild or late	129
Chronic ischaemic heart disease	e.g. homocystinuria; homozygous LDL receptor deficiency	71, 128
Nutritional deficiencies	e.g. selenium, thiamine	164, 161

Laboratory investigations
- Basic laboratory tests (*page 1*), repeat lactate, CK, ALT/SGOT, AST/SGPT
- Urine: simple tests, organic acids, glycosaminoglycans, oligosaccharides
- Vacuolated leukocytes
- Dried blood spots: acylcarnitines
- Serum: carnitine (free and total), CDG analysis; selenium, thiamine

Consider
- Leukocyte enzyme studies (incl. α-glucosidase [Pompe disease])
- Skin biopsy for enzyme studies
- Skeletal muscle biopsy in case of significant skeletal myopathy (histology, histochemistry, electron microscopy, biochemical and functional studies)
- Liver biopsy in case of significant hepatic dysfunction
- Exceptionally: endocardial biopsy (inflammatory changes, viral particles, signs of mitochondrial dysfunction, lysosomal storage, accumulation of lipids or glycogen)

Dysmorphic features

Most disorders of intermediary metabolism ("small molecule disorders") cause symptoms only after birth since metabolic homoeostasis is maintained via the placenta. Morphological abnormalities of prenatal (or postnatal) onset may be generated in metabolic disorders ...

... that affect structural macromolecules, such as peroxisomal disorders and congenital disorders of glycosylation;

... that cause progressive accumulation of metabolites, such as lysosomal disorders;

... that affect signalling pathways, such as the disorders of sterol synthesis;

... that affect cellular energy metabolism, such as pyruvate dehydrogenase deficiency.

Brain imaging may show structural abnormalities in many of these disorders, incl. disturbances of neuronal migration in peroxisomal disorders or cerebral malformations in mitochondrial disorders. In most disorders the disease course is progressive or dynamic, pointing to a metabolic process. However, some disorders such as the Smith-Lemli-Opitz syndrome may cause only mild dysmorphism and should be ruled out in all patients with intellectual disability and minor morphological anomalies (see *page 13*).

Peroxisomal disorders (page 143)
The most severe disorders of peroxisomal function (Zellweger syndrome) cause typical facial anomalies recognised at birth: High forehead, flat and broad base of the nose, epicanthus and abnormal ears. Skeletal abnormalities are most prominent in rhizomelic chondrodysplasia punctata.

Lysosomal storage disorders (page 129)
Apart from rare cases of non-immune fetal hydrops, children with lysosomal disorders often appear normal at birth (exceptions include I-cell disease). Morphological abnormalities develop over the first months and years of life, characterised by a typical ("coarse") facies, skeletal changes (dysostosis multiplex, short stature), changes of skin and hair and organomegaly.

Disorders of sterol synthesis (page 117)
Cholesterol plays an important role in the embryonal hedgehog signalling pathway. Disturbance of this pathway may be at least partly responsible for the typical congenital malformations seen in Smith-Lemli-Opitz syndrome (microcephaly, unusual facies, syndactyly of toes and genital anomalies in males) and other sterol synthesis disorders.

Disorders of energy metabolism (page 96)
Dysmorphism may be present at birth in mitochondrial disorders but is usually subtle and does not point to the diagnosis since other clinical features are more prominent. Children with severe PDH deficiency may resemble those with fetal alcohol syndrome.

Other disorders with morphological anomalies
• Menkes disease (*page 162*)
• Congenital disorders of glycosylation (*page 146*)
• Homocystinuria (*page 71*)

Investigations: see page 13, intellectual disability and dysmorphism

Liver disease

Manifestation patterns

Acute and chronic hepatocellular dysfunction may be associated with:
- Failure to thrive, muscle wasting, recurrent infections
- Encephalopathy: lethargy progressing to coma, behavioural changes, intellectual deterioration, pyramidal tract signs
- Bleeding disorder: haematemesis, epistaxis, haematoma
- Signs of portal hypertension: splenomegaly, ascites, shunt circulation
- Renal dysfunction – in several metabolic disorders this is due to toxins affecting both organs but renal dysfunction may also be the cause or the consequence of hepatic dysfunction

Hepatomegaly

Hepatomegaly may present as obvious abdominal distension or may be an incidental finding. Causes include increased cell size due to storage of various substances (e.g. fat, glycogen, lysosomal substrates, iron), inflammation/oedema, tumours (e.g. in tyrosinaemia type I), venous congestion or biliary obstruction.
- Consistency
  - Soft (e.g. glycogen storage disease)
  - Firm (e.g. lysosomal storage disease)
  - Hard and irregular (cirrhosis, e.g. in tyrosinaemia type I)
- Associated with splenomegaly?
  - Evidence of portal hypertension (cirrhosis) causing splenomegaly?
  - Evidence of generalised storage disorder? Liver cell function is normal in many lysosomal storage disorders.
  - Evidence of malignancy (leukaemia)?
- Evidence of metabolic disturbances or other abnormalities?
  - Hypoglycaemia (e.g. glycogen storage disease)
  - Renal disease (tyrosinaemia type I, Fanconi-Bickel disease)
  - Bleeding diathesis (tyrosinaemia type I)

Hepatomegaly may be a presenting feature in children with chronic hepatocellular dysfunction of various aetiologies (e.g. α_1-antitrypsin deficiency, Wilson disease).

Cholestasis

The usual presenting feature of cholestasis is jaundice or pruritus. It may be due to hepatocellular dysfunction or intrahepatic or extrahepatic obstruction of bile ducts. *Babies and infants with cholestasis require urgent referral to a specialist.* It may be associated with markedly increased serum cholesterol and xanthomata. Anicteric cholestasis or elevated transaminases and AP with normal GGT may be found in disorders of bile acid synthesis or secretion, as well as in conditions characterised by biliary hypoplasia, e.g. *Alagille syndrome. Cortisol deficiency* may present as cholestasis and hypoglycaemia.

Investigations (immunological and infectious causes not included)

General laboratory tests
- Routine laboratory tests incl. whole blood count, glucose, renal function tests, urea, creatinine, uric acid, CK, phosphate
- Basic metabolic laboratory tests (*page 1*)

Liver function tests
- Aminotransferases (ALT/SGOT, AST/SGPT) → hepatocellular injury
- Gamma-glutamyl transpeptidase (GGT) → cholestasis > hepatocellular injury
- Alkaline phosphatase (AP) → cholestasis
- Total bile acids → cholestasis
- Bilirubin (conjugated, unconjugated)
- Synthetic functions: albumin, prealbumin, coagulation studies, clotting factors (increased prothrombin time due to nutritional vit. K deficiency should be corrected within a few hours after vit. K administration)
- Lipid analyses: triglycerides, cholesterol

Additional investigations
- Amino acids (plasma) (*note*: elevated tyrosine may be found in hepatocellular dysfunction of any cause and does not necessarily indicate tyrosinaemia type I)
- Organic acids (urine) (specifically check for succinylacetone)
- Acylcarnitine profile (dried blood spot), carnitine status (serum)
- Galactose, Gal-1-phosphate, GALT activity
- Iron and ferritin
- Copper and coeruloplasmin (in children older than 4 yrs of age)
- α_1-Antitrypsin (α_1-AT) concentration and phenotype
- Sweat test (cystic fibrosis)
- α-fetoprotein (AFP)
- Bile acids, differentiated (urine)
- Consider CDG, lysosomal studies
- Consider coeliac disease (anti-gliadine and/or anti-endomysium antibodies, transglutaminase)

Differential diagnosis
- Hepatopathy after introduction of fructose → hereditary fructose intolerance
- Renal disease → galactosaemia, tyrosinaemia, hereditary fructose intolerance
- Storage disease → lysosomal/glycogen storage disorders
- Neuromuscular disease → peroxisomal/mitochondrial/glycogen storage disorders, CDG, Wilson disease
- Hemolytic anaemia → Wilson disease, fructose intolerance
- Cataract → galactosaemia, peroxisomal/lysosomal disorders, cerebrotendinous xanthomatosis
- Fetal hydrops (see *page 26*)

Neonatal liver failure

Disorder	Clinical features	Page
Mitochondrial hepatopathy, often mtDNA depletion	Muscular hypotonia, multi-system disease, encephalopathy, ↑ lactate	106
Neonatal haemochromatosis	Hepatocellular necrosis, cirrhosis; ↑↑ ferritin, ↑↑ AFP; transaminases may be low	164
Galactosaemia	Onset after milk feeds; jaundice, renal disease	82
Fatty acid oxidation disorders	(Cardio)myopathy, hypoglycaemia, ↑ lactate	91
Urea cycle disorders	↑↑ Ammonia	57
Niemann Pick type C	Jaundice, hypotonia, hepatosplenomegaly	138
Glycosylation disorders (CDG, e.g. type Ib)	Hepatomegaly, hepatocellular dysfunction, protein losing enteropathy, multi-system disease	146

Rarely: α_1-Antitrypsin deficiency, bile acid synthesis disorders

Severe neonatal jaundice

Disorder	Clinical features	Page
α_1-Antitrypsin deficiency	↓ α_1-Antitrypsin	
Niemann Pick type C	Hypotonia, hepatosplenomegaly	138
Galactosaemia	Onset after milk feeds; renal disease	82
Bile acid synthesis disorders	Cholestatic jaundice, malabsorption	120
Peroxisomal disorders (incl. Zellweger)	Severe hypotonia, areactivity, seizures, cataract, dysmorphic and skeletal abnormalities	143
Mevalonic aciduria	Hepatosplenomegaly, lymphadenopathy, anaemia	118
Tyrosinaemia type I	Severe coagulopathy, renal disease, ↑ AFP	68
Crigler-Najjar	Severe neonatal jaundice, kernicterus	
Rotor, Dubin-Johnson	Jaundice, normal liver function tests	
Progressive familial intrahepatic cholestasis (incl. Byler)	Cholestasis of hepatocellular origin; GGT may be normal	120
Alagille syndrome	Typical facies, other morphological anomalies	

Other causes: cystic fibrosis, hypothyroidism

Hepatomegaly + hypoglycaemia

Disorder	Clinical features	Page
Glycogen storage disease type I	Hepatocellular dysfunction, large kidneys, ↑↑↑ triglycerides, ↑ urate, ↑ lactate	83
Glycogen storage disease type III	Short stature, skeletal myopathy	84
Fanconi-Bickel disease	Tubulopathy, glucose/galactose intolerance	85
Disorders of gluconeogenesis	↑ Lactate	82
Glycosylation disorders (CDG, e.g. type Ib)	Hepatomegaly, hepatocellular dysfunction, protein losing enteropathy, multi-system disease	146

Other causes of neonatal hypoglycaemia (see *page 5*)

Hepatosplenomegaly in infancy

Disorder	Clinical features	Page
Lysosomal storage disease	Other symptoms and signs of generalised storage	129
Tangier disease	Polyneuropathy, orange tonsils, corneal clouding	127
Hepatic cirrhosis – α_1-Antitrypsin deficiency – Glycogen storage disease type IV – Tyrosinaemia type I		 84 68

Isolated *hepatomegaly* may be due to any disorder causing chronic hepatic dysfunction as well as a range of rare disorders. Isolated *splenomegaly* may be indicative of a lysosomal storage disorder (see *page 129*).

Infantile cholestatic jaundice

Disorder	Clinical features	Page
Hereditary fructose intolerance	Symptoms after fructose intake: hypoglycaemia, renal disease, failure to thrive, ↑ urate	81
Bile acid synthesis disorders	Cholestasis may be anicteric; malabsorption	120
Mitochondrial hepatopathy, e.g. mtDNA depletion syndromes, Pearson syndrome	Myopathy, multi-system disease, ↑ lactate	106
Progress. familial intrahepatic cholestasis (incl. Byler)	Pruritus, hepato(spleno)megaly, progessive cirrhosis; ↑ transaminases, ↑ AP, GGT may be normal!	120
Alagille syndrome	Typical facies, eye anomalies, cardiac defect, vertebral anomalies; dominant inheritance	

Infantile acute or chronic hepatic dysfunction

Disorder	Clinical features	Page
Mitochondrial hepatopathy, e.g. mtDNA depletion syndromes, Pearson syndrome	Myopathy, multi-system disease, ↑ lactate	*106, 108*
Glycosylation disorders (CDG, e.g. type Ib)	Hepatomegaly, hepatocellular dysfunction, protein losing enteropathy, multi-system disease	*146*
Tyrosinaemia type I	Jaundice, severe coagulopathy, renal disease, cirrhosis; ↑ AFP	*68*
Galactosaemia	Jaundice, failure to thrive, renal disease, cataract; later: cirrhosis	*82*
Fatty acid oxidation disorders incl. carnitine transporter deficiency	(Cardio)myopathy, hypoglycaemia	*91*

Reye-like syndrome (no jaundice) (see page 24)

Chronic hepatitis or cirrhosis in older children

Disorder	Clinical features	Page
Wilson disease	Neurological and renal disease, corneal ring	*162*
Haemochromatosis	Hepatomegaly, cardiomyopathy, diabetes mellitus, diabetes insipidus, hypogonadism	*163*
α_1-Antitrypsin deficiency	Failure to thrive; ↓ α_1-antitrypsin	
Tyrosinaemia type I	Coagulopathy, renal disease, ↑ AFP	*68*
Hereditary fructose intolerance	Symptoms after fructose intake: hypoglycaemia, renal disease, failure to thrive, ↑ urate	*81*
Transaldolase deficiency	Hepatosplenomegaly, cirrhosis (single patient)	*87*
Cystic fibrosis	Failure to thrive, recurrent airway infections	
Coelic disease	Failure to thrive, diarrhoea, small stature	

Reye-like syndrome

Reye syndrome is characterised by acute hepato-encephalopathy, usually complicating an infection. It is caused by acute mitochondrial dysfunction of varying aetiology. Reye syndrome in the narrow sense (caused by salicylates) has become rare. Inborn errors of metabolism are now the most likely cause of "Reye-like" syndrome.

Triggers: Salicylates, antiemetics, valproate, "idiopathic"
Clinical: Vomiting, lethargy, increasing confusion → coma, seizures, decerebration, respiratory arrest
Bioch.:   Hyperammonaemia, hypoglycaemia, metabolic acidosis, liver failure, ↑ fatty acids, dicarboxylic aciduria
Histol.:   Swollen hepatocytes, panlobular microvesicular fat deposition (steatosis); electron microscopy: "typical" mitochondrial abnormalities
Enzymes: Decreased activities of various mitochondrial enzymes, normal activities of cytosolic enzymes
DD: *Metabolic disorders*: urea cycle defects, fatty acid oxidation and ketogenesis defects, mitochondrial disorders, organic acidurias, gluconeogenesis defects, hereditary fructose intolerance
Diagn.:   Basic metabolic investigations, organic acids, orotic acid, carnitine status, acylcarnitines, amino acids in plasma and urine, basic mitochondrial studies. Consider additional biochemical, enzymatic or molecular studies.

Sudden unexpected death (in infancy)

Sudden infant death syndrome (SIDS) is defined as the sudden and unexpected death of a healthy child usually during sleep for which no cause is found by thorough autopsy. Using this strict definition, metabolic disorders are extremely unlikely to contribute to SIDS. *Metabolic disorders* (incl. fatty acid oxidation disorders, mitochondrial disorders, organic acidurias, gluconeogenesis disorders, fructose intolerance) have been found only in a small proportion of infants and children who died unexpectedly and who often had *previous clinical abnormalities* such as hypotonia, psychomotor retardation, seizures or hepatomegaly. Death may have been precipitated by gastroenteritis and these cases should not, by definition, be classified as SIDS. Given the low rate of autopsies performed on children who died unexpectedly in many countries, the following investigations may nevertheless be indicated, especially in countries where no extended newborn screening incl. long-chain fatty oxidation disorders is performed.

Investigations
- Forensic studies
- Basic post-mortem investigations (see *page 25*): organic acids (urine), amino acids (plasma, CSF), acylcarnitines (blood spots, bile, serum)
- Store EDTA blood and fibroblasts for specific mutation or enzyme enzyme studies, depending on the results of forensic studies (e.g. fatty liver) and basic investigations

Screening tests of *asymptomatic* siblings are unlikely to be productive if no specific diagnosis has been determined in the index case after adequate evaluation.

ALTE (acute life-threatening event)
An apparent life-threatening event (ALTE) is defined as an acute change in the breathing pattern of an infant with apnoea without respiratory efforts, sudden change of colour to pale or cyanotic, loss of muscle tone (rarely hypertonicity) or choking or gagging. By definition, the child is "resuscitated" from this situation by vigorous stimulation only. Metabolic investigations after a SIDS-like episode that is survived should include basic laboratory tests (*page 1*). Additional investigations such as acylcarnitines, amino acids (plasma), organic acids and mitochondrial studies should be considered in cases where the clinical history and/or basic laboratory findings suggest the possibility of an underlying metabolic disorder.

Post-mortem investigations

If a child dies of an unkown, possibly genetic disease, it is essential to collect representative post-mortem samples and discuss their analysis with a metabolic specialist. Without diagnosis, genetic counselling of the parents and reliable risk assessment for future children is not possible.

Samples
The following samples should be collected and stored for post-mortem analyses if a genetic disorder is suspected but specific metabolic investigations have not yet been performed:
- Serum and plasma (centrifuge several ml immediately, freeze in separate fractions)
- Dried blood spot (on filter paper card)
- Urine (freeze immediately – consider bladder wash with NaCl)
- Bile (spot on filter paper card for acylcarnitine analysis: bile contains particularly high levels of acylcarnitines and may be more useful than blood if available)
- DNA (3–10 ml EDTA whole blood, if necessary freeze without centrifuging)
- Culture fibroblasts (skin biopsy, may be obtained up to 24 hrs post mortem [or even later] and stored 1–2 days at ambient temperature in culture medium or 0.9% NaCl – do not freeze!)
- Consider CSF (several 1 ml fractions, freeze immediately, if possible at –70 °C)
- Consider vitreous fluid (freeze immediately)

Collect blood and urine samples prior to expected death.
Discuss investigations that may be indicated with the laboratory/metabolic specialist.

Biopsies
Fine needle biopsies should be considered before death since histological and enzymatic mitochondrial studies in post-mortem tissues are almost uninterpretable (if necessary, muscle biopsies may be obtained up to 1 hr post mortem). The acquisition of open organ biopsies (see *page 38*) depends on the clinical picture and is only indicated in exceptional cases. It should be discussed with the laboratory/metabolic specialist (samples are partly frozen immediately at –70°C or in liquid nitrogen, partly to be stored in glutaraldehyde for electron microscopy).
- Muscle (skeletal, consider heart): >500 mg (→ DNA, histochemistry, immuncytochemistry, analyses of energy metabolism; see *page 103*)
- Liver >200 mg (→ histochemistry, enzyme studies)

Basic investigations
- Amino acids in plasma (and CSF)
- Organic acids in urine
- Acylcarnitines from blood and/or bile spotted on a filter paper card
Note: Autolysis during the process of dying causes the intracellular fluid to mix with extracellular fluid. Huge misleading changes of plasma metabolites may be encountered.

Fetal hydrops

Fetal hydrops is the end stage of various conditions leading to the accumulation of fluid in fetal tissues and body cavities. It frequently affects the whole body but in some conditions may be restricted to certain compartments such as the abdomen (ascites). It is defined as "immune" (due to blood cell incompatibility) or "non-immune" and is most frequently caused by cardiovascular disease (up to 25% of cases), chromosomal disorders (> 10%), thoracic anomalies (up to 10%), anaemia (5–10%) and various other genetic and non-genetic condition. Inborn errors of metabolism are found only in a small proportion of cases. Metabolic investigations should be considered after detailed ultrasound examination, tests on maternal blood and invasive fetal testing (chromosomes, blood count, evidence of infection, haematological disorders, etc.) failed to reveal a diagnosis.

Metabolic disorders associated with fetal hydrops
- Lysosomal disorders
    - Mucopolysaccharidoses types VII (Sly), I, IVa
    - Sialidosis, mucolipidosis II (I-cell disease)
    - Sphingolipidoses (galactosialidosis, Niemann Pick A, Gaucher, Farber, GM_1 gangliosidosis, multiple sulphatase deficiency)
    - Lipid storage disorders (Niemann-Pick C, Wolman)
    - Sialic acid storage disease
- Sterol synthesis disorders
    - Smith-Lemli-Opitz syndrome, Greenberg dysplasia
    - Mevalonic aciduria
- Peroxisomal disorders (Zellweger)
- Glycogen storage disease type IV (Andersen)
- Glycosylation disorders (CDG)
- Congenital erythropoietic porphyria
- Primary carnitine deficiency
- Mitochondrial disorders, fumarase deficiency
- Neonatal haemochromatosis
- Any cause of severe cardiomyopathy

Unusual clinical observations

Urine and body odour

Odour	Substance	Disorder/origin
Animal-like, mouse-like	Phenylacetate	Untreated phenylketonuria, phenylbutyrate treatment
Maple syrup, "Maggi"	Sotolone	Maple syrup urine disease
Acrid (sweaty feet)	Isovaleric acid	Isovaleric aciduria, glutaric aciduria II
Male cat urine	3-OH-isovaleric acid	3-Methylcrotonylglycinuria, multiple carboxylase deficiency
Cabbage	2-OH-butyric acid	Tyrosinaemia type I
Rancid butter	2-Oxo-4-methiolbutyric acid	Tyrosinaemia type I
Sulphur	Hydrogen sulphide	Cystinuria
	Methionine	Tyrosinaemia type I, cirrhosis
Fish-like	Trimethylamine, dimethylglycine	Trimethylaminuria, dimethylglycinuria

Discolouration of urine or nappy/diaper

Colour	Substance	Disorder/origin	Confirmation
Brown or black	Homogentisic acid (may be pink/red)	Alkaptonuria	Urinary organic acids
	Met-haemoglobin	Myoglobinuria	Dipstick (see *page 16*, exercise intolerance)
	Haemoglobin	Haemoglobinuria	Dipstick, blood picture
	Melanin	Melanotic sarcoma	
Red	Erythrocytes	Haematuria	Microscopy
	Porphyrins	Porphyrias (not acute intermittent porphyria)	See *page 121*
	Various (most common)	Food colouring, red beet, blackberries, drugs (e.g. laxatives)	History
	External bacteria	Red diaper syndrome	Cloth nappies, > 24 hrs
Orange sand (or bright red)	Urate	Hyperuricosuria; physiological	Uric acid in blood and urine; see also *page 113*
Green-blue	Indigotin	Tryptophan malabsorption	Urine amino acids (Hartnup disease)
	Biliverdin	Obstructive jaundice	Serum bilirubin
	Methylene blue	Ingestion, treatment	History

Unusual laboratory findings

Unexpected findings in "routine" laboratory tests require critical evaluation. Particularly in patients with unusual and unexplained symptoms or clinical signs, they may be indicative of metabolic disease and can help to direct specific diagnostic investigations. The following table is not fully comprehensive.

Finding	Indicative of (selection)
Anaemia (macrocytic)	Disturbances in cobalamin and/or folic acid metabolism
Reticulocytosis	Glycolysis defects, disorders of the γ-glutamyl cycle
Vacuolised lymphocytes	Lysosomal storage disorders, juvenile NCL
↑ Alkaline phosphatase	Bile acid synthesis defects, hypoparathyroidism
↓ Alkaline phosphatase	Hypophosphatasia
↓ Cholesterol	Sterol synthesis defects, lipoprotein disorders, glycosylation disorders, peroxisomal disorders
↑ Triglycerides	Glycogen storage disorders, lipoprotein disorders
↑ CK	Dystrophinopathies, fatty acid oxidation disorders, glycogen storage disorders, glycolysis disorders, muscle AMP-deaminase deficiency, mitochondrial disorders
↓ Creatinine	Creatine synthesis disorders
↑ α-Fetoprotein (AFP)	Tyrosinaemia type I, hepatoblastoma, neonatal haemochromatosis, viral hepatitis, ataxia telangiectasia
↑ Uric acid	Glycogen storage disorders (incl. Fanconi-Bickel disease), fructose intolerance, disorders of purine metabolism, fatty acid oxidation defects, mitochondrial disorders
↓ Uric acid	Disorders of purine metabolism, molybdenum cofactor deficiency
↑ Iron, transferrin	Haemochromatosis, peroxisomal disorders
↑ Copper	Peroxisomal disorders, Wilson disease (urine, liver)
↓ Copper, coeruloplasmin	Wilson disease (serum), Menkes disease, acoeruloplasminaemia
Hypo(para)thyroidism	Mitochondrial disorders, CDG
Low CSF glucose	Glucose transport protein 1 (GLUT1) deficiency

Acanthocytosis

The appearance of spiculated erythrocytes in a peripheral blood smear or electron microscopy may be caused by changes in the lipid composition or structure of the red blood cell membrane. Two basic types are distinguished, *echinocytes* (burr cells) that have a serrated outline with small, uniform projections, and *acanthocytes* (spur cells) with few irregular spicules of varying size. Echinocytes and acanthocytes may be caused by a variety of conditions incl. advanced uraemia, severe hepatocellular damage, anorexia nervosa, hypothyroidism, vit. E deficiency or splenectomy; echinocytes are also common in (premature) neonates. Acanthocytes may be elicited by a *blood dilution test*: dilute patient and control samples 1:1 with normal saline, prepare smear, fix after 5 min – acanthocytosis is indicated by > 15% acanthocytes.

Differential diagnosis

Diagnosis	Clinical features	Age of onset	Page
Abetalipoprotein-aemia	Diarrhoea, fat malabsorption, vit. deficiencies, neurological abnormalities, ataxia, low cholesterol and triglycerides	Neonatal period	128
Wolman disease	Diarrhoea, failure to thrive, hepatosplenomegaly, adrenal calcifications	Neonatal period	142
Choreo-acanthocytosis	Progressive neurological symptoms, chorea, epilepsy, dementia;↑ CK, normal lipoproteins; *VPS13A* mutations	Adolescence or adult life	
McLeod phenotype, McLeod syndrome	Little or no reaction with various antisera in the Kell blood group system; somtimes progressive neurological symptoms, chorea;↑ CK, normal lipoproteins; *XK* mutations	Adult life (neurological symptoms)	

Special metabolic investigations are not required in ...

- Isolated moderate psychomotor delay
- Moderate failure to thrive
- Frequent infections
- Isolated delay in speech development in early childhood
- Occasional seizure, e.g. during fever, or a defined epileptic syndrome
- Healthy sibling of a previously asymptomatic infant who died of SIDS

An important factor in the evaluation of symptoms is their isolated appearance, i.e. the lack of additional neurological and/or systemic abnormalities.

Special metabolic investigations

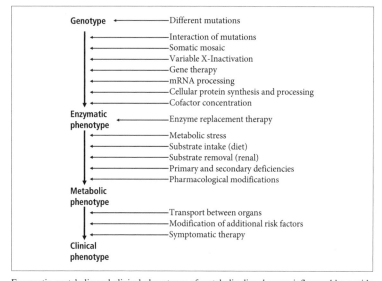

Enzymatic, metabolic and clinical phenotypes of metabolic disorders are influenced by a wide range of factors. The optimal level at which abnormalities can be recognised differs between disorders. Investigations should generally be as close as possible to the clinical phenotype: enzyme studies (when possible) are often more useful than molecular genetic studies. External factors that influence the concentrations of key metabolites (e.g. fasting, food intake) must be taken into consideration, and specific function tests may be required to identify diagnostic abnormalities.

Simple metabolic urine tests

These tests can rapidly provide initial clues, but have limited sensitivity and specificity. Their results therefore need to be viewed cautiously. If an inborn error of metabolism is considered, the investigation must not be limited to simple metabolic urine tests.

Dipstick test
Method: Test strip, with visual or automated evaluation
Detects: pH, glucose, acetoacetate, nitrite, bilirubin, urobilinogen, ketones …

Reducing substances in urine

Method: Test tablets (e.g. Clinitest®, Bayer)
Detects: Any reducing substances, particularly sugars

Substance	Disorder/origin
Galactose	Classical galactosaemia, galactokinase deficiency, severe liver disease (secondary galactose intolerance), Fanconi-Bickel disease
Fructose	Fructose intolerance, essential fructosuria
4-Hydroxyphenylpyruvate	Tyrosinaemia types I and II
Homogentisic acid	Alcaptonuria
Xylose, arabinose	Pentosuria, arabinosuria
Glucose	Diabetes mellitus, Fanconi syndrome
Oxalic acid (massive)	Hyperoxaluria
Salicylates, ascorbic acid	Drugs
Uric acid	Hyperuricosuria
Hippuric acid	Na-benzoate treatment of hyperammonaemia, malabsorption

Nitroprusside test (Brand reaction)

Method: 0.5 ml urine + 200 µl 5% Na-cyanide
Detects: Sulphur-containing acids (disulphides). False positive result may occur in severe ketosis, may be false negative in homocystinuria (assess total plasma homocysteine!).

Substance	Disorder/origin
Cystine	Cystinuria, hyperargininaemia, generalised hyperaminoaciduria
Homocystine	Classical homocystinuria, cobalamin deficiencies, cystathioninuria (bacterial in urinary tract infections)
Glutathione	Gammaglutamyl transaminase deficiency
Drugs	N-Acetylcysteine, penicillamine, captopril, ampicillin and others

Sulphite test

Method: Dipstick (e.g. Merckoquant® 10013, Merck), *fresh urine at the bedside*
Diagn.:   Sulphite oxidase and molybdenum cofactor deficiencies (particularly test early-onset epileptic encephalopathy). Positive result may be caused by various sulphite-containing drugs, false negative results may occur.

Amino acids (AA)

Amino acids are best analysed by ion exchange chromatography although individual amino acids can be reliably quantitated by tandem mass spectrometry.

Indications
- Selective metabolic screening (plasma)
- Hyperammonaemia (plasma + urine; if emergency phone laboratory!)
- Suspected aminoacidopathy (plasma; if emergency phone laboratory!)
- Suspected disorder of energy metabolism (plasma, metabolic profiling)
- Renal disorders – nephrolithiasis, Fanconi syndrome (plasma + urine)
- Positive nitroprusside test (urine, plasma [total homocysteine])
- Epileptic encephalopathy (plasma + CSF, obtain samples at the same time)
- Monitoring of protein restricted diet (plasma, 4 hrs fasting)

Samples
Blood: Minimum 0.5 ml plasma (EDTA, heparin) or serum (less preferable). Obtain sample in the morning (fasting) or approx. 4 hrs after last meal (prandial in newborns), centrifuge immediately and remove plasma/serum from the cell sediment. Ship on dry ice if possible; avoid shipping of non-centrifuged blood. Dried blood spot on filter paper card only allows assessment of selected amino acids; may be suitable for monitoring PKU patients. *Send emergency samples by courier (taxi).*

Urine: 5–10 ml, may be preserved with 2 drops of chloroform

CSF: Minimum 0.5 ml, send on dry ice. If blood-stained: unusable; if slightly blood-stained: centrifuge *and inform lab*! Always obtain and send plasma or serum sample in parallel (on dry ice).

Specific findings (plasma)
- ↑ Gln (+ Ala): hyperammonaemia; Gln/NH_3 < 1.6 µmol/µmol: transient neonatal hyperammonaemia; liver bypass
- Ile < 25 µmol/l: consider protein deficiency (adjust dietary intake if < 15)
- ↑ Ala, Pro; Ala/Lys ratio > 3: disturbance of energy metabolism (↑ pyruvate)
- Fischer ratio (Val + Leu + Ile)/(Phe + Tyr) < 2: liver failure with risk of hepatic encephalopathy
- ↑ Cit: renal disease

Caution
- Values depend on metabolic state (reference values 4–6 hrs after last meal):
  - Postprandial: ↑ essential AA (e.g. Lys, Phe, Tyr, Val, Leu, Ile, Gln, Cit)
  - Prolonged fasting: ↑ branched chain AA (Val, Leu, Ile); ↓ other AA
- Nonspecific changes (plasma):
  - Haemolysis, delayed centrifugation (> 20 min after sampling): ↓ Arg, Gln, Asn, Cys; ↑ Asp, Glu, Orn, Phe, Tyr, Tau, tHcy, etc.
  - Shipping at room temperature: ↓ Gln, Asn, Cys; ↑ Glu, Asp
- Tryptophan requires a special analytical method for true assessment, GABA and Hcy require special sample handling as well as special analytical methods (see below)
- Non-specific changes (serum): due to haemolysis/protein degradation during coagulation processes, serum concentrations are usually different from plasma concentrations

Total homocysteine (tHcy)

Blood should be centrifuged within 45 min to obtain EDTA or heparin plasma or serum. For exact measurement it is important to treat plasma or serum with a reducing agent that converts all Hcy species into the reduced form, HcyH, which is measured either directly or after derivatisation.

Normal values (fasting): children < 10 yrs: 3.5–9 μmol/l; > 10 yrs: 4.5–11 μmol/l; women premenopausal 6–15 μmol/l; post-menopausal 6–19 μmol/l; men 8–18 μmol/l.

Free GABA

Amino acid analysis determines total GABA, which is composed of physiologically active free GABA as well as variable amounts of homocarnosine. Only major elevations such as in GABA transaminase deficiency can be detected. To determine free GABA, plasma or CSF must be frozen immediately and shipped on dry ice (special analytical method).

Normal values: Plasma: 120–150 nmol/l

CSF: age < 1 yr: 20–40 nmol/l; > 1 yr: 20–150 nmol/l

Organic acids (OA)

Organic acids are analysed in urine, only in exceptional circumstances in other body fluids. The method of choice is gas chromatography-mass spectrometry (GC-MS); quantitation of specific OA is possible with stable isotope dilution assays.

Indications

If emergency phone laboratory!

- Unexplained metabolic crisis (metabolic acidosis, ↑ lactate, high anion gap, hypoglycaemia, ketonaemia, neonatal ketonuria, hyperammonaemia, cytopenia, etc.)
- Clincal features of systemic intoxication
- Suspected organic aciduria, aminoacidopathy
- Suspected fatty acid oxidation defect
- Suspected disorder of energy metabolism
- Unexplained hepatopathy
- Investigation of neurological or neuromuscular disorders
- Multi-system disorder, particularly in case of fluctuating/progressive symptoms

Special indications

(in specific/exceptional cases: discuss with laboratory)

- Quantitation of individual OA in urine/plasma for the exclusion of specific disorders or monitoring of therapy
- OA in CSF: "cerebral organic acidaemias"
- OA in plasma, CSF or vitreous fluid if no urine sample can be obtained, e.g. post mortem
- Separation of optical isomers (D,L-2-hydroxyglutaric acids; D,L-glyceric acids, D,L-lactic acids)

Samples

Urine: random (morning) sample (first available urine in cases of metabolic decompensation), 10 ml (volume depends on creatinine concentration: more urine required when creatinine level is low); (overnight) shipment at room temperature (recommended: preservation with 2–3 drops of chloroform or a few crystals of sodium azide) or preferably on dry ice (essential if succinylace-tone is to be determined)

Emergency samples by courier (taxi)!

Plasma, CSF, vitreous fluid: minimum 1.5 ml, freeze immediately, shipment on dry ice

Carnitine analyses

Acylcarnitine analysis by tandem mass spectrometry is the method of choice for the diagnosis of the classical organic acidurias and fatty acid oxidation disorders in neonatal and selective screen-ing. When coupled with amino acid analysis by tandem MS, it allows the rapid recognition of the majority of treatable metabolic disorders that present with acute crises. This method should there-fore be available for emergency analyses in all metabolic centres. Long-term acylcarnitine mon-itoring may be useful for some disorders. Acylcarnitine analysis may miss the carnitine transport-er defect for which exact determination of *free and total carnitine* (*carnitine status*) in serum and urine is necessary. The carnitine status is also used for monitoring carnitine treatment as quanti-fication by tandem MS is not usually sufficiently accurate.

Free carnitine and acylcarnitines (differentiation)

Indic.: Newborn screening; diagnosis of organic acidurias or fatty acid oxidation disorders; hypoglycaemia, monitoring of treatment

Method: Electrospray tandem MS or fast atom bombardment tandem MS

Sample: Dried blood spot (filter paper card: newborn screening card, "Guthrie" card), plasma/serum, urine, bile

Findings: Diagnostic elevation of specific acylcarnitines (see *pages 51–53*)

Carnitine status (total carnitine, free carnitine, acylcarnitine)

Indic.: Suspected disorder of intermediary metabolism with accumulation of CoA-esters, pri-mary and secondary carnitine deficiency, monitoring of treatment

Method: Radiochemical

Sample: 1 ml serum or plasma; 5 ml urine

| | Carnitine | | | Acylcarnitine differentiation (dried blood) |
	Total	Free	Acyl-bound	
Fasting	n	↓	↑	
CT deficiency	↓↓	↓↓↓	↓↓	↓ All carnitines
CPT1 deficiency		n–↑	↓↓	↓ C_{16}–$C_{18:1}$
CACT/CPT2 deficiency[1]; FAO disorders[2]	n–↓	↓	↑	Specific (but not 100% sensitive)
Single organic acidurias[3]	↓		↑	Specific
Respiratory chain disorders	n–↓	n–↓	n–↓	n

[1] Suspected CACT/CPT2 deficiency: analyse acylcarnitines in plasma. [2] *Note*: carnitine analyses are generally normal in mitochondrial HMG-CoA synthase deficiency. [3] Only few organic acid-urias (acylcarnitine analyses cannot replace organic acid analysis); CT = carnitine transporter; CPT = carnitine palmitoyltransferase; CAC = carnitine acylcarnitine carrier; FAO = fatty acid ox-idation.

Other special metabolic investigations

International quality control networks (e.g. ERNDIM/CAP) have been established for various special metabolic investigations incl. amino acids and organic acids. However, participation is generally voluntary (enquire with laboratory).

Bile acids

Indic.: Suspected bile acid synthesis defect (see *page 120*), peroxisomal disorder (see *page 143*)

Method: FAB-(fast atom bombardment)-MS/GC-MS, electrospray tandem MS

Sample: 5 ml urine or 2 ml bile fluid

Free fatty acids (FFA) and 3-hydroxybutyrate

Indic.: Hypoglycaemia, fasting test

Method: Photometric

Sample: 1 ml serum/plasma, shipment on dry ice (to avoid lipolysis)

Normal: *Non-fasting*: FFA and 3-hydroxybutyrate low (< 300 µmol/l)

Fasting: both elevated up to 3–4 mmol/l (see *page 167*)

Galactose (Gal) and galactose metabolites

Indic.: Suspected disorder of galactose metabolism (see *page 81*); see also *page 49* (newborn screening)

Method: Variable, discuss with laboratory

Sample: Dried blood spots for galactose concentration und enzyme studies (fluoride/EDTA blood is also suitable for galactose determination). EDTA/heparin whole blood for Gal-1-phosphate, enzyme studies, DNA studies; consider plasma für galactose, urine for galactitol.

Discuss with laboratory; if in doubt store dried blood spots + 2 ml EDTA whole blood at room temperature (up to 48 hrs).

Findings: – Galactose (plasma, dried blood spots); pathological if > 10 mg/dl (0.55 mM)

– Galactose-1-phosphate (erythrocytes); pathological if > 0.5 mg/dl (19 µM)

– Galactitol (urine); pathological if > 10 mmol/mol creatinine

– Enzyme studies (erythrocytes): GALT, galactokinase, epimerase

– Mutation studies (EDTA whole blood)

Glutathione and metabolites

Indic.: Suspected disorder of the γ-glutamyl cycle (see *page 77*)

Method: HPLC

Sample: Washed erythrocytes from 3 ml EDTA whole blood; enquire about sample processing with the laboratory

Glycosylation studies (CDG analysis)
Indic.:   Suspected disorder of protein glycosylation, CDG (see *page 146*)
Method: Transferrin electrophoresis/isoelectric focusing, HPLC, MS-MS, capillary electro-
            phoresis
Sample: 0.5–1 ml serum (plasma unsuitable)
Findings: Different subtypes correspond to different enzyme deficiencies; abnormal glycosyla-
            tion patterns (secondary changes) also in alcoholism, galactosaemia, fructose intoler-
            ance, hepatitis C, etc.

Lysosomal studies
Glycosaminoglycans (GAG; mucopolysaccharides)
Indic.:   Suspected lysosomal storage disease/mucopolysaccharidosis (see *page 133*)
Method: Screening: GAG quantitation ("DMB test")
            Specific analysis: electrophoretic separation of different GAGs
Sample: 10–20 ml urine without additives
Findings: GAG elevation – may be absent/borderline in MPS III (Sanfilippo) and IV (Morquio)
            but differentiation by electrophoresis can identify the pathological excretion of hepa-
            ran/keratan sulphate and is therefore always recommended

Oligosaccharides, free neuraminic acid (sialic acid)
Indic.:   Suspected lysosomal storage disease/oligosaccharidosis (see *page 135*)
Method: Thin-layer chromatography with various staining reagents
Sample: 10–20 ml urine, shipment frozen or preserved with 2–3 drops of chloroform
Findings: Reliable diagnosis of: GM_1 and GM_2 gangliosidoses, α-mannosidosis and β-mannosi-
            dosis, fucosidosis, Gaucher disease, sialic acid storage disease, sialidosis, aspartyl-
            glycosaminuria; may also be abnormal in Pompe disease

Orotic acid
Indic.:   Suspected heterozygous OTC deficiency, urea cycle defects, disorders of pyrimidine
            metabolism, mitochondrial disorders, allopurinol test
Method: HPLC, MS-MS, capillary electrophoresis
Sample: 5 ml urine
Findings: Elevation indicates increased production of mitochondrial carbamyl phosphate (urea
            cycle disorders; see *page 57*) or disorder of pyrimidine metabolism; unexplained ele-
            vations also in other disorders, e.g. Rett syndrome, Lesch-Nyhan syndrome, "benign
            orotic aciduria"

Peroxisomal studies
Very long-chain fatty acids (VLCFA), phytanic acid, pristanic acid
Indic.:   Suspected peroxisomal disorder (see *page 143*)
Method: GC-MS
Sample: 1 ml plasma
Findings: Specific elevations of fatty acids that are metabolised in the peroxisomes

Plasmalogens
Indic.:   Suspected peroxisomal disorder (see *page 143*)
Method: GC-MS
Sample: Erythrocytes (EDTA whole blood)
Findings: Reduced in rhizomelic chondrodysplasia punctata and peroxisome biogenesis disorders

Porphyrins

Indic.:   Suspected porphyria (see *page 121*); tyrosinaemia type I (see *page 68*); screening tests for porphobilinogen in urine (Hoesch test, Watson-Schwartz test) where acute hepatic porphyria is suspected

Sample: Random urine sample (20 ml), faeces (approx. 5 ml), heparinised whole blood (5–10 ml), store in a cool and *dark* place, ship without additives

Pterins

Indic.:   Hyperphenylalaninaemia, BH_4 test, suspected neurotransmitter defect

Method: HPLC

Sample: Urine (5 ml) serum or CSF (1 ml); keep in a dark place (dark urine collection bag), centifuge blood immediately, freeze all samples immediately, ship on dry ice (sample preparation for shipping without dry ice: check with lab)

Findings: Specific elevations or reductions of neopterin or biopterin

Purines and Pyrimidines

Indic.:   Suspected disorder of purine or pyrimidine metabolism (see *page 112*); life threatening side-effects of pyrimidine antimetabolites, i.e. pharmacogenetic complications

Method: HPLC, GC-MS (dihydropyrimidines), MS-MS, capillary electrophoresis

Sample: 5 ml urine (preferably morning sample) or 24 h urine collection (keep in a cool and dark place), ship frozen (particularly important for the diagnosis of adenylosuccinase deficiency), otherwise overnight shipment, recommended preservation with 2–3 drops of chloroform/10 ml (do not acidify); record medication; for further modalities see *page 113*

Pyruvate

Indic.:   Pyruvate should not be routinely measured as values obtained may be spurious and lactate is the more relevant and reliable test. Pyruvate is sometimes used to determine the lactate/pyruvate ratio. Never measure pyruvate without lactate. Most samples for pyruvate analysis are only suitable for in-house analysis.

Method: Photometric

Sample: Perchloric acid extraction (ask lab)

Normal: Blood: 50–100 µmol/l; CSF: 70–140 µmol/l; lactate/pyruvate ratio: <20 (elevated in respiratory chain disorders, typically normal in PDH deficiency)

Serotonin

Indic.:   Suspected disorder of biogenic amine metabolism; carcinoid syndrome

Method: HPLC

Sample: 2 ml EDTA whole blood + 6 mg ascorbic acid, freeze immediately at –70°C, ship on dry ice

Sterol biosynthesis intermediates
Indic.:   Suspected disorder of cholesterol biosynthesis, e.g. Smith-Lemli-Opitz syndrome (see
            page 124), cerebrotendinous xanthomatosis (*page 120*)
Method: GC-MS
Sample: 1 ml plasma

Trimethylamine (TMA)
Indic.:   Malodour, suspected trimethylaminuria (see *page 165*)
Method: Headspace GC; NMR spectroscopy
Sample: Random urine sample, acidify with HCl, send by express mail or on dry ice
Findings: ↑ Free TMA or ↓ TMA-oxide (normal > 90% of total TMA)

Biopsies and enzyme studies
Obtain local protocols and discuss modalities with laboratory/pathology before the samples are
obtained.

Leukocytes
• 5–10 ml heparinised whole blood, shipment at ambient temperature within 24 hrs

Skin biopsy (fibroblasts)
• In culture medium → fibroblasts (do not freeze!)
• Formalin → histology
• Consider samples in glutaraldehyde (electron microscopy)

Conjunctival biopsy
• Formalin → histology

Liver biopsy
• Formalin → histology
• Consider samples in glutaraldehyde (electron microscopy)
• Consider samples for biochemical evaluation and enzyme studies: freeze immediately in liq-
  uid nitrogen

Muscle biopsy *(see also page 103)*
• Thin muscle fibre in 2% glutaraldehyde (electron microscopy)
• Several pieces of muscle fibre frozen immediately in liquid nitrogen (for histology 1 cm length
  with recognisable fibre structure), store at –70°C, for enzyme histochemistry and immunohis-
  tochemistry, biochemical evaluation, enzymes studies, mutation analysis as indicated
• Immediate isolation of mitochondria for investigations in native tissue
• Small piece for formalin fixation and paraffin preparation (do not freeze) for light microscopy

Molecular genetic investigations

Indications
- Primary diagnosis or confirmation of diagnosis, particularly in disorders in which a biochemical or enzymatic diagnosis is not possible, not reliable or requires invasive procedures (e.g. organ-specific disease expression, disorders of structural, receptor or membrane proteins)
- To obtain information on the course of disease and prognosis and the potential value of specific treatment options in disorders with established genotype-phenotype correlations
- Prenatal diagnosis and family studies in genetic counselling

General considerations

Are mutation studies necessary?
Enzyme studies or other functional (phenotypic) investigations, if available, may be more (cost) effective for reaching a diagnosis or for an assessment of disease severity and other characteristics of the deficient protein. On the other hand, mutation analyses may be the diagnostic method of choice when biochemical findings are inconsistent or unreliable, when functional tests are tedious, unpleasant or potentially dangerous, or when the enzyme is not expressed in a convenient tissue, such as in heterozygous OTC deficiency, hereditary fructose intolerance, glycogen storage disease type I or HMG-CoA synthase deficiency. Identification of previously characterised mutations may allow rapid assessment of functional parameters such as disease severity or BH_4 responsivity in PKU.

Costs of mutation studies
Remuneration of diagnostic mutation analyses differs markedly between countries. Costs often depend on the number of exons (or genes) that require sequencing; it may be advisable to enquire about costs with the laboratory before tests are ordered.

Quality of mutation studies
Quality control schemes for DNA sequencing consistently show an error rate of at least 1% even in expert laboratories, and many labs do not provide an adequate clinical interpretation of the molecular results. If the results do not fit the clinical picture it may be justified to repeat the test. Mutation analyses should be carried out in accredited (or certified) diagnostic labs run by qualified human (molecular) geneticists. It is advisable to choose labs that are familiar with inborn errors of metabolism and have excellent knowledge of the respective gene and its variants as well as genotype-phenotype correlations.

How unlikely is the diagnosis when no mutation is found?
Sequencing of all coding exons and adjacent introns, possibly in conjunction with screening for large deletions and duplications (e.g. by multiple ligation-dependent probe amplification, MLPA), is able to detect >95% of disease-causing mutations in most metabolic disorders. Nevertheless, negative molecular results do not usually rule out a diagnosis. DNA analysis reports in this situation should include information on the sensitivity of the methodology.

Rules and pitfalls (recessive disorders)
- Mutation screening, i. e. testing for a few known common mutations in a gene, is relatively inexpensive and suitable for some conditions such as MCAD deficiency, LCHAD deficiency or hereditary fructose intolerance. However, it is important to take the origin of the patient into consideration since the frequency of mutations differs markedly between populations.

- Identification of a single heterozygous mutation generally supports the diagnosis, assuming that the method used failed to identify the second mutation. However, simple (coincidental) carrier status cannot usually be excluded.
- A normal result without any putative mutation argues against the diagnosis provided that a highly sensitive method has been employed and the parents of the affected child are unrelated (non-consanguineous).
- Novel mutations should be interpreted with caution as effects on protein function or pre-mRNA splicing may be difficult to predict with certainty.
- Identification of two heterozygous mutations: inheritance in trans (on different chromosomes) should normally be confirmed through analysis of both parents (beware of non-paternity).
- Premature termination of the analyses when two (novel) mutations have been found may be unwise as there could be additional (and more relevant) mutations in the gene.
- Apparent homozygosity of a point mutation may be due to heterozygosity for this mutation and a large deletion on the other allele. This phenomenon can be recognised through analysis of both parents.
- Additional caveats: Is the clinical picture fully explained by the genetic findings? Is the disorder fully penetrant? Could there be additional, non-genetic factors of pathogenesis?

Novel molecular genetic approaches
Some patients may be expected to have an aut. rec. inborn error of metabolism, but clinical and metabolic findings may not be specific enough to suggest a candidate gene for sequencing. Novel genome-wide methods such as SNP-array genotyping are helpful in some of these cases.
- Autozygosity mapping in patients with consanguineous parents allows the identification of homozygous genomic regions that trace back to the same ancestor through both parents. The disease gene is expected to be in one of these regions, and candidate genes may be recognised through assessment of adequate databases. Sequence analysis of genes outside such regions is generally not indicated.
- Linkage analyses are possible if there are two or more affected siblings in a family. Methodology and interpretation resemble autozygosity mapping but there are usually more candidate regions if the parents are unrelated.
- Genome sequencing is successfully combined with autozygosity mapping or linkage analysis for the identification of novel diseases on a research basis. The analysis is often restricted to the exons of all known genes (exome sequencing). Sensitivity is still limited since only 90–95% of all exons may be covered in adequate depth, and correct interpretation of novel variants identified may be a challenge. The possibility of incidental findings should be discussed before the analyses.

> Mutation analyses in children should only be performed if there is an important medical consequence *in childhood*. Carrier analyses in healthy siblings of children with metabolic disorders are not indicated and should not be carried out even when requested by the parents. The results of mutation studies should be explained to the patient (or his/her family) through full genetic counselling.

Sample
5–10 ml *EDTA whole blood* (or less), do not separate cells, shipment by ordinary mail (within 24 hrs) or if frozen on dry ice (enquire with laboratory).
If no blood sample available: *filter paper card, biopsies, fibroblasts, etc.*

Function tests

Many metabolic disorders are best recognised through metabolic profiling, i.e. repeated measurement of appropriate metabolites (glucose, lactate, amino acids, etc.) throughout day (and night). This approach is also used to assess the response to external factors and to monitor and tailor treatment. Rapid advances in enzymatic, molecular and other diagnostic techniques permit an increasing number of diagnoses to be obtained without tests of tolerance. Sometimes controlled function tests are required to show that a patient responds abnormally to specific metabolic challenge.

Metabolic profiling

Indications
- Evaluation of substrate metabolism (mitochondriopathies, disorders of glycogen homoeostasis)
- Evaluation of nitrogen disposal (urea cycle disorders)
- Hypoglycaemia of unknown cause
- Monitoring of treatment, e.g. assessment of glucose homoeostasis and catabolism in disorders with reduced fasting tolerance

Procedure
- Obtain a fasting urine sample and blood samples before breakfast in the morning:
    - Glucose, lactate, alanine (amino acids)
    - Consider acylcarnitines, free fatty acids, 3-hydroxybutyrate
    - Consider ammonia
    - Store serum sample for additional analyses
    - Urine: test strip; consider organic acids and orotic acid
- Obtain blood samples before and one hr after each meal throughout the day:
    - Glucose, lactate, consider amino acids (Ala) and ammonia; store serum sample
- Consider one blood sample during the night
    - Glucose, lactate, amino acids (Ala); store serum sample
Other parameters may be included depending on clinical features and suspected disorders.

Interpretation
- Hypoglycaemia <2.6 μmol/l (<45 mg/dl) (see *page 5*)
- A possible mitochondrial disorder or pyruvate dehydrogenase deficiency (see *page 96*) may be indicated by:
    - Postprandial elevation of lactate (>2.1 mmol/l) or rise >20%
    - Paradoxical postprandial ketosis
    - Postprandial elevation of alanine >(600–700 μmol/l), alanine/lysine ratio >3
- Normalisation of elevated lactate in preprandial/fasting sample: consider pyruvate dehydrogenase deficiency
- Preprandial hypoglycaemia, variable elevation of lactate: consider glycogen storage diseases
- Postprandial elevation of ammonia, glutamine or orotic acid: consider mild variant of urea cylce disorder

Protein challenge

The test is particularly useful in the diagnosis of mitochondrial disorders which show a pathological postprandial increase of lactate, alanine and other small amino acids. It may also show impaired detoxification of ammonia but should not usually be used for the diagnosis of urea cycle disorders as it may trigger acute hyperammonaemia.

Procedure

- Preprandial blood sample; measure blood gases, blood sugar, amino acids, lactate, ammonia, ketones
- Normal meal enriched with protein and sugar = total amount of 1 g/kg BW each of protein and carbohydrate/sugar
- Postprandial blood sample 90 min after meal; same analyses as above; postprandial urine collected for 2 hrs; measure lactate, organic acids, orotic acid

Interpretation

Lactate should not rise by ≥ 20% from baseline and remain < 2.1 mmol/l. NH_3 should remain normal (< 100 μmol/l). Acid-base status should be normal. Alanine should stay < 600–700 μmol/l, with an alanine/lysine ratio of < 3.

Glucose challenge

Glucose is catabolised to pyruvate which enters mitochondrial energy metabolism (see *page 96*). Mitochondrial disorders occasionally show a significant elevation of lactate only after substrate (glucose) challenge. *Glucose challenge is contraindicated* when lactate has been consistently elevated or when a significant postprandial increase of lactate has been demonstrated during metabolic profiling. In these cases, appropriate enzyme studies (muscle biopsy) and possible molecular analyses should be undertaken upon completion of the basic biochemical analyses.

Indications

- Suspected mitochondrial disorder but apparently normal lactate values
- Suspected glycogen synthase deficiency (hepatomegaly should be excluded)
- Suspected glycogen storage disease, normal mutation/enzyme studies (patient should have recurrent preprandial hypoglycaemia with elevated lactate, glucose should be low normal at beginning of test)

Procedure

Before commencing test

- Complete basic investigations incl. repeated blood lactate, urinary organic acids, alanine (plasma amino acids), etc.
- Glucose challenge should be carried out in the morning after overnight fasting (younger infants: > 4–5 hrs after last meal)

At start of test
- Secure i.v. access
- Collect base-line blood samples, measure lactate, glucose, acid-base status
- Give glucose 2 g/kg (max. 50 g) as special drink or 10% oral solution (store in fridge – more palatable when chilled), consider nasogastric tube in small children (flush with water)
- Collect blood samples after 30, 60, 90, 120, 180 min: measure lactate, glucose, acid-base status; collect urine for 2 hrs, analyse organic acids, lactate

Interpretation

Lactate should not rise >20% and should not reach pathological values (>2.1 mmol/l). Acid-base status and urine analyses should remain normal. Glucose levels should rise and remain within the normal range. A marked elevation of lactate may indicate a mitochondrial disorder which, however, is not excluded by a normal result. An excessive rise of glucose and lactate may indicate glycogen synthetase deficiency (GSD0). An inappropriate increase of glucose and decrease of lactate may indicate Fanconi-Bickel disease. A fall of lactate after glucose challenge may indicate glycogen storage disease type I.

Prolonged fasting test

The response to fasting is altered in many inborn errors of metabolism incl. hormonal disorders, disorders of gluconeogenesis, glycogenolysis and fatty acid utilisation. Affected children may be asymptomatic and may show normal laboratory results until they become ill or metabolically stressed. Assessment of metabolic changes in response to fasting may be helpful in cases in which extensive investigations have failed to lead to the diagnosis. Controlled fasting is also used to determine a safe fasting tolerance to tailor therapy in individual patients, e.g. in patients with long-chain fatty acid oxidation disorders. A fasting test is rarely indicated before the age of 6 mths.

> *Caution*: In some patients fasting can lead to the production of toxic metabolites and severe, sometimes fatal complications. *It is essential to complete metabolic profiling* incl. repeated acylcarnitine analyses (dried blood spots) *and other metabolic investigations* incl. functional or molecular analyses prior to a fasting test.
> **In general, fasting tests for metabolic disorders should only be performed in specialist metabolic units and only after other, less risky investigations have been completed without a clear diagnosis.**

Indications
- Recurrent documented hypoglycaemia of unknown cause
- Assessment of fasting tolerance
- Suspected impaired fatty acid oxidation after extensive, comprehensive metabolic work-up has remained inconclusive
- Reye-like disease (after analysis of acylcarnitines and organic acids)
- Lactic acidosis
- Recurrent cyclic vomiting
- Recurrent episodes of symptomatic ketonuria

Procedure

Before commencing test

- Complete other metabolic investigations incl. metabolic profiling; obtain normal results for carnitine status, organic acids, acylcarnitines and, where indicated, other special investigations/tests. Fasting tests should be avoided for the diagnosis of fatty acid oxidation disorders; as far as possible these should be excluded prior to fasting.
- Stable metabolic state for > 2 mths; normal diet for this patient, good nutritional state
- Obtain informed consent from the parents (sequelae of hypoglycaemia, e.g. seizure)
- The maximum duration of the fast should be decided before starting and will be determined from the history (expected fasting tolerance) and the age of the child. Unless otherwise directed, this should be as follows:

Age	< 6 mths	6–8 mths	8–12 mths	1–2 yrs	2–7 yrs	> 7 yrs
Length	8 hrs	12 hrs	16 hrs	18 hrs	20 hrs	24 hrs

- The fast should be timed so that there is negligible risk of clinical symptoms before 8:00 a.m. and blood specimens can be collected during the working day.
- In special circumstances (e.g. suspected fructose-1,6-biphosphatase deficiency) prepare glucagon test for the end of fasting.
- Prepare an individual test form for recording clinical data and laboratory results

At start of test

- An indwelling cannula should be in place throughout the test, both to collect the blood samples without difficulty and to give i.v. glucose if necessary. The test has to be stopped if the line is lost.
- Carefully record the time when the fast started and when samples were taken. This is essential for interpretation.
- The child's clinical condition must be watched carefully. Document in the notes how well the fast is tolerated and the clinical state at the end of the fast.
- If the child is thirsty plain water may be given and this should be encouraged.

Samples

- Start of fast:
  - Bedside glucose
  - Laboratory blood glucose, blood gases
  - Store additional serum sample
  - Urinary organic acids, ketones (test strip)

From the first missed feed onwards (usually 8:00 a.m.), laboratory blood glucose (or bedside glucose) should be measured *hourly* so as to identify hypoglycaemia without delay. All urine passed should be checked for ketones. Store serum samples for possible additional investigations every time a venous blood samples is taken. Carefully label all samples immediately and freeze if necessary. Pyruvate and acetoacetate are *not* routinely measured as these samples require deproteinisation at the bedside.

- 8:00 a.m. blood tests:
  - Bedside glucose
  - Laboratory blood glucose, blood gases, lactate
  - Consider free fatty acids, 3-hydroxybutyrate
  - Store additional serum sample

- End of fast blood tests:
  - Bedside glucose
  - Laboratory blood glucose, blood gases, lactate
  - Free fatty acids, 3-hydroxybutyrate
  - Insulin, cortisol, growth hormone
  - Carnitine status, acylcarnitines
  - Amino acids
  - Store additional serum sample
- Collect first urine sample after end of fast:
  - Organic acids
  - Ketones (test strip)
  - Store part of the urine sample

Terminate fasting if:

- **Hypoglycaemia < 2.6 μmol/l (< 45 mg/dl), or clinical symptoms such as irritability, sweating and drowsiness**
- **Metabolic acidosis (bicarbonate < 15 mmol/l)**
- Collect end-of-fast samples, ask laboratory for an urgent blood glucose result on this sample. The end-of-fast specimens should still be collected if the child has a fit although the lactate value may be falsely elevated.
- If the child is symptomatic: give i.v. glucose 0.2 g/kg (**2 ml/kg of 10% dextrose, prepared beforehand**) as a slow bolus
- If the child is still symptomatic after the bolus: check bedside glucose; only give more glucose if glucose is low (< 3 mmol/l) as too much CAN BE HARMFUL!
  Suitable infusion: 5–8 mg/kg/min (3–5 ml/kg/hr of 10% dextrose)
- If the child is asymptomatic: give a carbohydrate drink followed by something to eat
- Before discharging a child after the test, a meal should be seen to have been eaten and tolerated by the child

Interpretation

Hypoglycaemia below 2.6 mmol/l or symptoms of reduced consiousness are abnormal until proven otherwise; for interpretation see also *page 5*. Blood concentrations of free fatty acids (FFA) and subsequently 3-hydroxybutyrate rise during the test; high concentrations of FFA but an insufficient increase in 3-hydroxybutyrate (see *page 167* for normal values) indicate a disorder of fatty acid oxidation or ketogenesis. Blood lactate concentrations should remain below 2 mmol/l but may be falsely elevated if the child is struggling. Hypoglycaemia with elevated lactate and ketosis may be found in glycogen storage or gluconeogenesis disorders and mitochondrial disorders. Elevated alloisoleucine (plasma amino acids) is indicative of (intermittent) maple syrup urine disease. Hyperinsulinism should be suspected if plasma insulin is not completely suppressed at the time of hypoglycaemia (see *page 88*), whilst plasma cortisol below 400 nmol/l may indicate adrenocortical insufficiency.

Glucagon test

The glucagon test examines the availability of glycogen for compensation of low blood glucose. It has been largely superseded by enzyme or mutation studies but may be useful in some circumstances.

Indications
* Confirmation of a glycogen storage disorder
* Confirmation of depleted glycogen stores at the end of a fasting test, indicative of disorders of gluconeogenesis
* Assessment of glycogen stores in neonatal hypoglycaemia and suspected congenital hyperinsulinism

Test requirements
Low blood glucose <3.5 mmol/l (<60 mg/dl) at baseline; the patient should remain fasting unless there are symptoms of hypoglycaemia or blood glucose decreases further.

Procedure
* Base-line blood glucose
* Give 500 μg (or 30–100 μg/kg) glucagon i.m.
* Blood glucose after 15, 30, 45 and 60 min
* Include analysis of blood lactate when a glycogen storage disease is a possibility.

Interpretation
Blood glucose should rise by more than 1.4 mmol/l (25 mg/dl) within 45 min. An insufficient rise indicates depleted glycogen stores or inability to convert glycogen into glucose. This may be observed in *disorders of gluconeogenesis* (e.g. fructose-1,6-biphosphatase deficiency) at the end of a fasting test. The same is true for Fanconi-Bickel disease. Blood glucose remains low but lactate increseases in *glycogen storage diseases*. There is a normal increase of blood glucose in *congenital hyperinsulinism*.

Tetrahydrobiopterin (BH$_4$) test

BH$_4$ is a cofactor of phenylalanine hydroxylase (PAH) and other hydroxylases (see also *page 153*). Administration of BH$_4$ in individuals with hyperphenylalaninaemia leads to a reduction of plasma Phe concentrations when there is either a primary disorder of BH$_4$ metabolism or a cofactor-sensitive form of phenylketonuria (PKU).

Indications
* Rapid diagnosis of BH$_4$ cofactor deficiency (i.e. a pterin defect, see *page 153*) in children with hyperphenylalaninaemia detected by newborn screening.
* Identification of BH$_4$ sensitivity in children with PKU (PAH deficiency). The proposed loading test for sapropterin dihydrochloride (Kuvan®) involves re-assessment of the diet, measurement of Phe tolerance and titration of therapy in responders to treatment.

Test requirements
* Blood Phe >600 μmol/l (400 μmol/l for neonates with possible cofactor deficiency)
* Combination with Phe loading prior to BH$_4$ administration is not recommended as results are difficult to interpret (are likely to be false positive)
* Constant protein intake during the test
* No acute disease

Procedure
Neonates (possible cofactor deficiency)
- Obtain baseline blood for Phe + Tyr analysis and urine for pterin analysis (*page 37*)
- Give 20 mg/kg sapropterin/BH$_4$ diluted in water 30 min before normal meal
- Obtain blood samples after 1, 2, 4, 8 + 24 hrs, collect urine for 4–8 hrs (must be protected from light)

Older patients with PKU

Day 1:	• No sapropterin/BH$_4$
	• Blood for Phe + Tyr at T0, T8, T16 and T24 (= T0 day 2)
Day 2:	• Sapropterin/BH$_4$ 20 mg/kg BW (orally with food)
	• Blood for Phe + Tyr + biopterin at T0, T8, T16 and T24 (= T0 day 3)
Day 3:	• Sapropterin/BH$_4$ 20 mg/kg BW (orally with food)
	• Blood for Phe + Tyr + biopterin at T0, T8, T16 and T24

Interpretation
- Phe reduction of more than 80–90% after 4–8 hours is highly indicative of BH$_4$ deficiency. In BH$_4$-deficient patients there is a simultaneous increase in Tyr levels also starting 4 hours after sapropterin/BH$_4$ administration.
- Test is considered positive for BH$_4$ sensitivity in children with PKU (PAH deficiency) if blood Phe is at least 30% below baseline at T16/T24 on days 2 and 3. As a rule, some reduction of blood Phe should already be noted after 8 hours.
- Reduction of blood Phe by 30% at T8 but less than 30% at T16 or T24 indicates non-responsiveness.
- The loading test must be positive on day 3. A positive test on day 2 but not on day 3 indicates non-responsiveness.
- In ambiguous cases (e.g. reduction of blood Phe just under 30% on day 3) an extended 1-week loading test may be completed, with the same amount of sapropterin/BH4 and the same sampling protocols.
- Blood collection protocol can be modified to only one (T24) or two (T16 and T24) time points in a trial of 1–2 wks.
- Failure to respond after 1–2 wks indicates non-responsiveness.

Phenylalanine loading test
The Phe loading test investigates the hydroxylation capacity of Phe to Tyr, thereby examining the function of the enzyme phenylalanine hydroxylase as well as the availability of the cofactor BH$_4$. Relevant for interpretation are the respective readings of Phe, Tyr and pterins after Phe challenge.

Indications
- Undiagnosed dystonic movement disorder, suspected Segawa syndrome
- Suspected disorder of biogenic amine or pterin metabolism (see *page 151*)

Procedure
The test should be carried out at least 1 hr after a light breakfast. No food until the end of the test.
- Obtain blood sample for baseline values
- Give 100 mg/kg L-phenylalanine in orange juice, if necessary through nasogastric tube
- Obtain blood samples after 1, 2, 4 and 6 hrs

Samples

Approx. 2 × 1 ml EDTA/heparin blood at each time point, centrifuge and freeze plasma immediately (two portions of 0.5 ml), ship on dry ice (alternatively dried blood spots; consult laboratory). Analyse Phe, Tyr, pterins.

Interpretation

A slow decrease of Phe and a delayed increase of Tyr indicate reduced hydroxylation capacity. If biopterin rises sufficiently, a defect of pterin metabolism is excluded and the defect lies in phenylalanine hydroxylase, e.g. heterozygosity for PKU. Evaluation must utilise age-specific cut-off values.

Allopurinol test

The allopurinol test detects increased throughput in pyrimidine synthesis (see *page 115*), e.g. due to increased carbamylphosphate production from mitochondrial detoxification of ammonia (see *page 57*).

Indication

Suspected heterozygous or mild ornithine transcarbamylase deficiency.
- Unclear transient or intermittent hyperammonaemia with neurological symptoms (e.g. epilepsy, ataxia)
- Unclear comatose or encephalopathic episodes, neurodegenerative disorders in girls
- Females at risk of OTC deficiency when mutation cannot be identified in propositus

Procedure

Avoid caffeine (decaffeinated coffee is acceptable), tea, cocoa, chocolate, cola, benzoate-containing beverages 24 hrs before test. Women should be 7–12 days after their last menstrual period if possible. The test is usually started in the morning.
- Basal values: collect urine sample
- Give oral allopurinol: 100 mg (< 6 yrs), 200 mg (6–10 yrs), 300 mg (> 10 yrs)
- Collect urine in 4 fractions: 0–6 hrs, 7–12 hrs, 13–18 hrs, 19–24 hrs

Samples

Obtain 10 ml of each urine fraction, freeze and send frozen, or conserve with 3 drops of chloroform and send by express mail. Label sample tubes accurately, inform laboratory of all medication taken on the preceding days. Quantification of orotic acid and orotidine should be done by HPLC (rather than by a colorimetric method; see *page 36*).

Interpretation

Excessive increase of orotic acid and orotidine indicates increased throughput in pyrimidine synthesis. The test has only a moderate sensitivity and specificity, and test results may be false positive or false negative. A negative allopurinol test (or protein challenge) does not exclude heterozygous OTC deficiency as mosaicism in the liver (lyonisation) may be skewed in favour of normal hepatocytes to a degree that renders the detection of metabolic effects impossible. If in doubt, consider mutation analysis or liver biopsy (enzyme analysis).

Newborn screening

Newborn population screening was introduced in the 1960s for the detection of phenylketonuria and was later extended to a few other disorders. In the mid 1990s, tandem mass spectrometry (MS-MS) for the identification of acylcarnitines, amino acids and various other metabolites was shown to allow *extended newborn screening* and was consecutively incorporated into screening programmes woldwide. MS-MS enables the diagnosis and treatment of a much larger number of metabolic disorders (fatty acid oxididation disorders, organic acidurias, some urea cycle defects, additional disorders of amino acid metabolism) in all newborns. Whilst this is of obvious benefit e.g. in severe medium-chain acyl-CoA deficiency and glutaric aciduria type I, it has also led to the identification of many children with mild biochemical abnormalities or disease variants of doubtful clinical relevance. In consequence, newborn screening by tandem MS may lead to unnecessary treatment of healthy children as well as undue anxiety of parents. Today there are great differences between the panel of disorders screened for, partly because there is no consensus on the basic decision criteria for inclusion. Whereas US programmes analyse and report all possible disorders and biochemical abnormalities, European programmes are much more restricted. Guidelines and fact sheets are available for follow-up and confirmatory diagnostics after a positive NBS result (*USA*: www.acmg.net, resources; *UK*: http://newbornbloodspot.screening.nhs.uk).

Disorders detected by newborn screening
- Most programmes: phenylketonuria, hypothyroidism
- Regional variation: galactosaemia, biotinidase deficiency, maple syrup urine disease, adrenogenital syndrome, cystic fibrosis, sickle cell anaemia, thalassaemias
- Extended programmes: MS-MS incl. aminoacidopathies, organic acidurias, fatty acid oxidation disorders, some urea cycle defects

Newborn screening for inborn errors of metabolism

Here we list disorders or metabolites covered by newborn screening programmes. The consequences of positive screening results differ between conditions. Sometimes only a repeat analysis from a second screening card is required. In other cases immediate initiation of therapeutic measures is necessary which may require referral to a specialised metabolic centre. Management advice in the text is intended for asymptomatic patients and should obviously be adjusted if the child has symptoms. Parents may need to understand that urgent intervention is necessary even though newborn screening also detects asymptomatic variants of many conditions. In all conditions, the diagnosis can be confirmed by mutation studies (often genotype-phenotype correlations). "Urgent admission/consultation" = within 1–2 days. "Immediate admission/consultation" = immediate evaluation of the neonate by or in close co-operation with a paediatric metabolic specialist/endocrinologist.

Note: In most instances it is not necessary to stop breast-feeding (see individual diseases for details).

Abbreviations: Metab. = key metabolites, Confirm. = confirmatory studies, Comm'ts = additional comments, AA = amino acids, OA = organic acids, DBS = dried blood spot (repeat screening card), DC = dicarboxylic acid.

Phenylketonuria (PKU; *page 67*)
Metab.:   ↑ Phe, ↓ Tyr, ↑ Phe/Tyr ratio
Confirm.: AA plasma; exclude cofactor deficiency (*page 153*): pterines in urine, DHPR activity in DBS (*page 35*); consider BH_4 test (*page 46*)

Variants: PKU = severe form requiring treatment; MHP = no treatment required
DD: Prematurity, liver disease/hepatic failure, parenteral nutrition; ↑ Phe + ↑ Tyr: tyrosin-
           aemia type 2 or 3, transient hypertyrosinaemia (premature neonates)
Advice: Urgent hospital admission/outpatient assessment; continue breast feeding

Galactosaemia *(page 82)*
Method: Gal-1-P uridyltransferase (GALT) activity; quantitation of galactose (Gal) and Gal-
           1-P (either in parallel or as second tier tests; in GALT and UDP-Gal epimerase [GALE]
           deficiencies almost all galactose [>90%] is Gal-1-P).
DD: ↓ GALT activity: classical galactosaemia (GALT deficiency)
           ↑ Gal: inborn errors of Gal metabolism (see *page 81*: GALT/GALE/GALK deficien-
           cies); liver failure (various causes); open ductus venosus arantii
Caution: GALT activity may be false normal after erythrocyte (exchange) transfusion. Exposure
           of test card to humid heat may cause denaturation of enzymes and consecutively a
           false positive result for GALT activity.
Advice: (neonate on regular formula/breast milk):
           Galactose (total) < *50 mg/dl* (1.7–2.2 mM): immediate outpatient assessment of gen-
           eral condition, liver function (coagulation! INR), confirmatory studies; commence lac-
           tose-free formula if any impairment, final decision about diet when results of confir-
           matory studies are available
           Galactose (total) > *50 mg/dl* (2.2 mM): **immediate** hospital admission and lactose-
           free formula; assess general condition, thorough assessment of liver and renal func-
           tion (coagulation! INR), confirmatory studies
Confirm.: Specific investigations *(page 35)*: galactose, galactose-1-phosphate, GALT activity;
           mutation studies (common mutations in Europeans, Duarte variants)

> Make sure that appropriate blood samples are obtained at the start of a lactose-free diet. If in
> doubt: store filter paper card with dried blood spots. Diagnosis of classical galactosaemia by
> measuring GALT activity can be pursued also after start of diet.

Biotinidase deficiency *(page 158)*
Method: Determination of biotinidase activity (% normal); residual activity <10% = severe de-
           ficiency, 10–20(–30)% = partial deficiency
Caution: Exposure of test card to humid heat may cause denaturation of enzymes and consec-
           utively a false positive result
Advice: Urgent metabolic consultation; severe deficiency: start biotin 10 mg/day; otherwise
           wait for confirmation
Confirm.: Biotinidase analysis in serum/plasma

Maple syrup urine disease *(page 66)*
Metab.:   ↑ XLE (= Leu + Ile + Allo-Ile + OH-Pro), ↑ Val, ↑ XLE/Ala
DD: Total parenteral nutrition, hydroxyprolinaemia *(page 75*, probably non-disease)
Advice: **Immediate** hospital admission, stop protein, i.v. glucose
Confirm.: AA plasma (Allo-Ile)

Tyrosinaemia type I *(page 68)*

Metab.: Succinylacetone, ↑ Tyr (less specific and sensitive)
DD: Elevated tyrosine (normal succinylacetone): hepatic failure, tyrosinaemia types 2 and 3, transient hypertyrosinaemia (mainly premature neonates)
Advice: **Immediate** hospital admission, stop protein, i.v. glucose
Confirm.: AA plasma, OA (urine: succinylacetone)

Homocystinuria *(page 71)*

Metab.: ↑ Hcy; more common: ↑ Met (2nd tier Hcy from DBS, where available)
DD: Liver failure (↑ Met and Tyr); MAT I/III (↑ Met only)
Advice: Urgent hospital admission/outpatient assessment; continue breast feeding
Confirm.: AA plasma, Hcy

Elevation of other amino acids

Citrulline: DD: citrullinaemia (see *page 59*): ↑ Cit; argininosuccinic aciduria (see *page 59*): ↑ Cit, ↑ Asa
Advice: **immediate** hospital admission, stop protein, check NH_3, i.v. glucose
Confirmation: AA plasma and urine
Arginine: Argininaemia *(page 59*; low sensitivity, Arg frequently normal in newborns)
Advice: urgent hospital admission/outpatient assessment, check NH_3; continue breast feeding
Confirmation: AA plasma and urine
Glycine: Non-ketotic hyperglycinaemia (see *page 74*)
Advice: urgent hospital admission/outpatient assessment; continue breast feeding
Confirmation: AA plasma (if symptomatic: plasma + CSF)

Elevated long-chain acylcarnitines

DD: ↑ C_{16}, C_{18}; low C_0: carnitine translocase or CPT2 deficiency *(page 92)*
↑ $C_{14:1}$, C_{14}, $C_{14:1}/C_4$, $C_{14:1}/C_{12:1}$, etc.: VLCAD deficiency *(page 93)*
↑ $C_{16}OH$, $C_{18:1}OH$ LCHAD/MTP deficiency *(page 93)*
Advice: **Immediate** hospital admission, stop protein, i.v. glucose
Confirm.: Acylcarnitines (plasma), OA (urine), carnitine status

Elevated medium-chain acylcarnitines

Diagn.: MCAD deficiency (see *page 93*): ↑ C_8, C_8/C_2, C_8/C_{12}
Advice: Urgent metabolic consultation
Confirm.: Acylcarnitines (plasma), OA (urine)

Elevated C_5 (C_5/C_2)

DD: Isovaleric aciduria *(page 63)*, 2-methylbutyric aciduria *(page 65*; possibly non-disease)
Advice: **Immediate** hospital assessment:
Child unwell, acidosis → admission, stop protein, i.v. glucose, L-carnitine
Child well → confirmatory diagnostics, continue breast feeding
Confirm.: Acylcarnitines plasma, OA urine

Elevated C$_5$OH

DD: Multiple carboxylase deficiency (*page 159*)
          HMG-CoA lyase deficiency (*page 94*), also ↑ C$_6$DC
          3-Methylcrotonylglycinuria (*page 63*; possibly non-disease)
          3-Methylglutaconic aciduria I (*page 63*; probably non-disease in childhood)
          3-Oxothiolase deficiency (see *page 95*), also ↑ C$_{5:1}$
Advice: **Immediate** hospital assessment:
          Child unwell, acidosis → admission, stop protein, i.v. glucose, L-carnitine
          Child well → confirmatory diagnostics, continue breast feeding
Confirm.: Acylcarnitines plasma, OA urine

Elevated C$_4$

DD: SCAD deficiency (*page 94*), IBD deficiency (*page 65*)
Advice: Probably non-diseases (→ C$_4$-acylcarnitine is excluded from NBS programmes in several countries): outpatient assessment, continue breast feeding
Confirm.: Acylcarnitines (plasma), OA (urine)

Elevated C$_3$ (C$_3$/C$_0$, C$_3$/C$_2$, C$_4$DC)

DD: Propionic aciduria (*page 62*); methylmalonic aciduria (*page 62*); cobalamin disorders (*page 156*); many false positive cases
Advice: **Immediate** hospital assessment:
          Child unwell, acidosis → admission, stop protein, i.v. glucose, L-carnitine
          Child well → confirmatory diagnostics, continue breast feeding
Confirm.: Acylcarnitines (plasma), OA (urine)

Elevated C$_0$

Diagn.:   CPT1 deficiency (*page 92*): ↑ C$_0$/(C$_{16}$ + C$_{18}$)
Confirm.: Acylcarnitines (plasma), carnitine status
Advice: Urgent hospital admission

Very low C$_0$

DD: Carnitine transporter deficiency (*page 92*); organic acidurias, prematurity; if FTR normal: test mother for carnitine deficiency
Advice: Urgent metabolic consultation
Confirm.: OA urine, carnitine status, fractional tubular re-absorption (FTR) of carnitine

Elevation of multiple acylcarnitines (C$_4$ – C$_{18}$)

Diagn.:   Multiple acyl-CoA dehydrogenase deficiency (see *page 94*)
Advice: **Immediate** hospital assessment
Confirm.: Acylcarnitines (plasma), OA (urine)

Glutaric aciduria I *(page 62)*

Metab.:   ↑ C$_5$DC (= glutaryl-CoA)
Advice: Urgent hospital admission
Confirm.: Acylcarnitines plasma, OA urine

Malonic aciduria *(page 65)*
Metab.:   ↑ C_3DC, C_4DC
Advice: Urgent hospital admission
Confirm.:   Acylcarnitines in plasma, methylmalonic acid in plasma

Newborn screening for non-metabolic disorders

Congenital hypothyroidism
Primary hypothyroidism is mostly caused by non-genetic causes that disrupt normal thyroid development. Secondary or tertiary hypothyroidism is much less common (pituitary or hypothalamic dysfunction; TSH not elevated, requires direct assay of T_4).
Method: ↑ TSH (and/or ↓ T_4) (note cut-off differences between labs)
Confirm.:   TSH, FT_4 and T_3 resin uptake in plasma (take sample before treatment)
Advice: TSH elevation >20 µU/ml: urgent assessment, await confirmatory tests; >50 µU/ml: **immediate** assessment and start of L-thyoxine (50 µg for full-term infants)

Congenital adrenal hypoplasia
Mostly 21-hydroxylase deficiency (CYP21B gene) → deficiency of glucocorticoids and mineralocorticoids, excess androgens
Clinical: *Severe form*: salt wasting, vomiting, lethargy (hyperkalaemia, hyponatraemia), *females*: congenital virilisation; *males*: scrotal hyperpigmentation; mild forms
Method: ↑ 17-OH-progesterone (ELISA)); beware: up to 1% false positive
Confirm.:   17-OHP in plasma, steroid profile in blood or urine
Advice: **Immediate** assessment; check electrolytes, blood sugar; careful re-evaluation of genitalia; in case of abnormalities start hormone replacement with hydrocortisone and mineralocorticoids

Metabolic pathways and their disorders

Amino acid and peptide metabolism

Deficiencies of enzymes involved in amino acid metabolism frequently result in accumulation of toxic substances and subsequent organ damage. The brain, liver and kidneys are the most frequently affected organs. Acute symptoms are often associated with catabolic states that lead to the breakdown of endogenous proteins and the release of large amounts of amino acids. The clinical features result from the toxicity of the accumulating metabolites and concurrent product deficiency; they depend on the severity of the enzyme deficiency and the extent of protein intake or endogenous amino acid release in protein catabolism. Some disorders cause chronic neurological damage without acute decompensation. Many disorders of this group are recognised by newborn screening with tandem MS (*page 49*). Most *aminoacidopathies* are caused by deficiencies of cytosolic enzymes and are recognised by amino acid analysis in plasma (or urine). The classic *organic acidurias* are caused by deficiencies of mitochondrial enzymes required for the (beta-oxidative) breakdown of coenzyme A-(CoA-)activated small carbonic acids (after deamination of amino acids) and are diagnosed by the analysis of urinary organic acids. Organic acidurias frequently disturb energy metabolism and cause metabolic (lactic) acidosis. Treatment usually involves (a) protein restriction, (b) supplementation of amino acids with unimpaired metabolism as well as trace elements, and (c) specific measures for detoxification if indicated. Treatment is not restricted to childhood but usually must be continued throughout life.

Typical presenting features
- Acute coma/ataxia/encephalopathy without evidence of encephalitis
- Acute, unclear deterioration or prolonged disease course of a non-specific infection
- Progressive neurological symptoms
- Multi-system disorder
- Unexplained acidosis
- Ketonuria in the neonate
- Hyperammonaemia

Age of presentation
Disorders of amino acid metabolism can present at any age but are not usually symptomatic at birth or on the first day of life. Disorders with acute presentation often present at times of protein catabolism, e.g. in the *neonatal period* (metabolic transition, delayed food intake), *late infancy* (change to protein-rich meals with greater intervals; common infections with fever, vomiting and reduced food intake) or *puberty* (changes in growth rate, psychosocial factors).

Principles of treatment

This section explains general rules for treatment once the diagnosis is known. See *page 3* for the management of children with metabolic decompensation of unknown cause and *page 7* for the emergency treatment of hyperammonaemia.

In disorders with acute presentation, increased protein breakdown while in a catabolic state (fasting, infection, vaccination, surgery) may cause the accumulation of large amounts of toxic metabolites in a very short time, leading to severe CNS damage or death. In such disorders it is imperative to interrupt a catabolic state at an early stage of impending decompensation. As this usually happens at home, it is essential to educate the family about how to react adequately to the metabolic state.

Patients should carry an *emergency card* or bracelet containing essential information and phone numbers as well as instructions on emergency measures. *Vaccinations* should be carried out as recommended and should include vaccinations against varicella, hepatitis A and influenza. Special precautions must be taken before and after *surgery*.

Principles of long-term treatment

1. *Diet*: Protein restriction plus a semisynthetic amino acid supplement that does not contain the accumulating amino acids (or precursor amino acids of accumulating toxins); supplementation of minerals and trace elements. Beware of protein deficiency due to "overtreatment" – may cause protein catabolism (may be recognised by plasma amino acid analysis).
2. If indicated give *specific detoxifying drugs*, e.g. in urea cycle defects
3. If indicated give *specific vitamins or cofactors*, e.g. in biotinidase deficiency and holocarboxylase synthetase deficiency, vit. B_6- or B_{12}-responsive homocysteinaemias, vit. B_{12}-responsive methylmalonic acidurias, vit. B_2-responsive multiple acyl-CoA dehydrogenase deficiency
4. Give *carnitine* (50–100 mg/kg/day) in all disorders that cause intramitochondrial accumulation of CoA esters, i.e. most organic acidurias (caution if a long-chain fatty acid oxidation disorder is a possible DD)
5. *Monitor growth* regularly: weight, size, head circumference, development
6. Regular *laboratory monitoring* of patients on protein-restricted diets (metabolic parameters depend on the disease): blood count, calcium, phosphate, magnesium, iron, liver and kidney function tests, alkaline phosphatase, total protein, albumin, pre-albumin, cholesterol, triglycerides, vitamins, carnitine, acid-base status, ammonia, lactate, amino acids in plasma, organic acids in urine, acylcarnitines

Treatment of intercurrent illness at home

In order to prevent metabolic decompensation during intercurrent illness with poor feeding, vomiting, fever, etc.:

- Stop protein intake, give sufficient fluid (water, tea) and calories (carbohydrates as glucose polymers/maltodextrin) with some salt every two hours, according to the following table (Dixon & Leonard, *Arch Dis Child* 1992):

Age	Glucose polymer/maltodextrin solution		
	%	kcal/100 ml	Daily volume
0–1 yrs	10	40	150–200 ml/kg
1–2 yrs	15	60	95 ml/kg
2–10 yrs	20	80	1,200–2,000 ml/day
>10 yrs	25	100	2,000 ml/day

- Start adding protein after 24–48 hrs at the latest: one day half the normal amount of protein, one day ¾, then the full amount of normal protein
- Assess nutritional state one week after the illness (plasma amino acids). There may be a transient increase in protein requirement after an intercurrent illness.

Immediate hospital admission and i.v. treatment is indicated when vomiting persists, fluid and dextrose intake remain poor, the clinical condition deteriorates or the disease course is prolonged. When presenting in an emergency clinic these patients must be assessed by a specialist immediately and further treatment initiated without delay.

Emergency treatment in the hospital

Every person with a known disorder of amino acid metabolism and the possibility of acute decompensation should be attached to a hospital with a dedicated team of metabolic specialists that can be reached at any time. For holiday trips it is prudent to enquire about metabolic services in the respective region.

1. Take *appropriate blood samples*: basic laboratory tests (*page 1*), amino acids in plasma, liver and renal function tests, etc.
2. *Interrupt a catabolic state* by high-dose energy substitution: 10% glucose infusion, 150 ml/kg/day (~10 mg/kg/min, ~60 kcal/kg/day) (exceptionally via nasogastric tube), add i.v. insulin if necessary (check lactate); add parenteral lipids 1 g/kg/day
3. *Stop protein intake*: The accumulation of toxic metabolites in some organic acidurias can be reduced by intestinal antibiotics (metronidazole, colistine).
4. *Ensure adequate fluid and electrolyte intake*: aim for a sodium concentration ≥ 140 mmol/l to reduce the risk of cerebral oedema
5. *Start antibiotics* if there is any suggestion of an infectious cause
6. *Carry out detoxifying measures* depending on the disease and laboratory findings: increased diuresis, dialysis, haemofiltration
7. *Consider specific drug treatment* (vitamins, carnitine, carbamylglutamate, etc.) depending on the disease and laboratory findings

Age-dependent glucose requirement (mg/kg body weight/minute)

Age	0–12 mths	1–3 yrs	3–6 yrs	6–12 yrs	Adolescents	Adults
Glucose	7–9	6–8	6–7	5–6	5	3–4

Glucose production rate y (mg/min) = $0.0014x^3 - 0.214x^2 + 10.411x - 9.084$ (x = weight in kg)

Urea cycle disorders and inherited hyperammonaemias

Urea cycle defects are among the most common inborn errors of metabolism (cumulative incidence approx. 1:8,000). They can present at all ages, are usually easy to diagnose (but frequently overlooked) and in principle treatable. The emergency analysis of blood ammonia must be part of the basic investigations in all patients with unclear encephalopathy at at any age.

Biochemistry

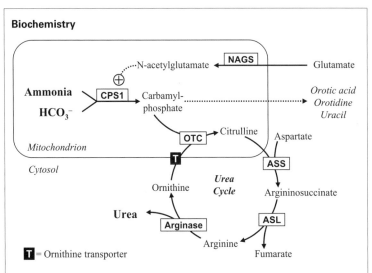

= Ornithine transporter

Ammonia (NH_3) arising from amino acid metabolism is detoxified mainly through its conversion to urea in the liver. The enzyme catalysing the inital condensation of ammonia and bicarbonate, *carbamylphosphate synthase I* (CPS1), requires activation by N-acetylglutamate which itself is formed by *N-acetylglutamate synthase* (NAGS). Carbamylphosphate is subsequently bound to ornithine by *ornithine transcarbamylase* (OTC). Citrulline is formed, transported out of the mitochondrion and bound to aspartate by *argininosuccinate synthase* (ASS) (aspartate in this reaction is provided by the mitochondrial transporter citrin which is part of the malate-aspartate shuttle also required for the recycling of cytosolic NADH). The resulting argininosuccinate is split by *argininosuccinate lyase* (ASL) into fumarate and arginine which in turn is hydrolysed by *arginase* into ornithine and urea. Urea, as a harmless carrier of two N-residues, is excreted in the urine; ornithine is transported back into the mitochondrion by the *ornithine transporter*, thus completing the urea cycle.

Hepatic NH_3 detoxification is additionally effected (in low capacity) through the action of *glutamine synthase* at the perivenous part of the hepatic lobule. The enzyme adds an amino group to glutamate and thus gives glutamine a buffer function. An increased glutamine concentration in plasma (normal <700 µmol/l) is the most sensitive indicator of insufficient urea synthesis. A liver bypass (e.g. open ductus venosus in the neonate) causes hyperammonaemia with insufficient formation of both urea and glutamine. Insufficient arginine intake (e.g. parenteral nutrition) or transport defects involving the dibasic amino acids cause a deficiency of intramitochondrial ornithine, accumulation of carbamyl phosphate and hyperammonaemia.

Clinical features

- *Neonates*: rapidly progressive symptoms in the first days of life after a short symptom-free interval: lethargy, poor feeding, hyperventilation, seizures, progressive encephalopathy with deepening coma, temperature instability, loss of reflexes, intracranial haemorrhages due to coagulation defect (check by ultrasound)
- *Infants and children*: failure to thrive, feeding problems, vomiting, chronic neurological symptoms, episodic encephalopathy with lethargy, ataxia, seizures
- *Adolescents and adults*: chronic neurological or psychiatric symptoms, behavioural problems, episodes of disorientation, lethargy, psychosis, recurrent encephalopathy usually associated with high protein intake, catabolism or stress

Acute management

See page 7. The most urgent laboratory parameter is blood ammonia. Hyperammonaemia is one of the most urgent emergencies in metabolic medicine and must be treated immediately and aggressively.

Long-term treatment

1. *Maintain anabolic state*
2. *Limit protein intake*: if possible provide minimal requirements as natural protein; if necessary replace natural protein (contains approx. 50% essential amino acids) by half the amount of an essential AA mixture
3. *Give arginine* 100–200 mg/kg/day (OTC/CPS deficiency) or up to 600 mg/kg/day (ASS/ASL deficiency). Citrulline (same dose) should be given instead of arginine in severe OTC/CPS deficiency (eliminates an additional ammonium group).
4. *Remove ammonia*: Na-benzoate 250–400 mg/kg/day oral (elimination of 1 mol NH_3 per mol of glycine) and/or Na-phenylbutyrate 250–500 mg/kg/day oral (elimination of 2 mol NH_3 per mol of glutamine)
5. *Give vitamins and trace elements* (e.g. folic acid 500 µg/day)
6. *Consider lactulose* 3 × 4–20 g/day (binds intestinal ammonia due to acid pH) or (intermittent) non-absorbable antibiotics
7. *Consider liver transplantation*

Monitor laboratory values frequently and adjust diet to avoid excessive protein reduction (overtreatment). Target values:

- *NH_3* < 80 µmol/l
- *Orotic acid* < 10 mmol/mol creatinine (defects beyond CPS)
- *Gln* < 800(–1,000) µmol/l (should not be too low during Na-phenylbutyrate therapy)
- *Gly* 100–150 µmol/l (during Na-benzoate therapy)
- *Arg* 80–150 µmol/l (if too low increase the dose of arginine/citrulline)
- *Essential AA* should all be in the normal range, particularly during Na-phenylbutyrate therapy; specific target values: Ile > 15 µmol/l (marker of sufficient protein intake), Thr > 100 µmol/l (> 70 in the 1st yr; marker of long-term exogenous protein intake, may be elevated in plasma after a period of protein deficiency)
- *Avoid hypokalaemia* during Na-phenylbutyrate or Na-benzoate therapy (check regularly)

Sufficient fluid intake (> 1,000 ml/day)
Vaccinations as recommended, plus vaccinations against varicella, hepatitis A, influenca
Treat infections early, if necessary "blindly" with antibiotics
Avoid hidden nitrogen, e.g. liquorice (salmiac)

Carbamylphosphate synthase I (CPS1) deficiency

Clinical: Often severe neonatal disease; milder variants occur at any age
Diagn.:   AA (plasma): ↑ Gln, ↓–n Cit, Arg; normal or low orotic acid (urine); enzyme studies: liver

Ornithine transcarbamylase (OTC) deficiency

Clinical: *Males*: usually severe hyperammonaemia (lethal in the neonate); milder variants not uncommon
            Females: clinical picture variable even within a family, dependent on the X-inactivation pattern in the liver; severe symptoms/encephalopathy in 15–20%
Genetics: X-chromosomal; *OTC* gene
Incidence: 1:14,000 (most common urea cycle defect)
Diagn.:   AA (plasma): ↑ Gln, ↓ Cit, Arg (↑ Lys due to shortage of 2-oxoglutarate); ↑↑ orotic acid/uracil (urine); mutation analysis is method of choice for diagnosis in females, allopurinol test if appropriate (see *page 48*); enzyme studies: liver

Citrullinaemia type I

Clinical: Often milder course with manifestation after the neonatal period
Enzyme: Argininosuccinate synthase; *ASS* gene
Diagn.:   AA (plasma): ↑↑ Cit, ↓ Arg; ↑ orotic acid (urine); enzyme studies: fibroblasts

Argininosuccinic aciduria

Clinical: Neurological and hepatic problems (liver fibrosis) despite good control of NH_3 levels with sufficient arginine intake (detoxification of one molecule of NH_3 via argininosuccinic acid); hair abnormalities (trichorrhexis nodosa)
Enzyme: Argininosuccinate lyase; *ASL* gene
Diagn.:   AA (plasma, urine): ↑↑ argininosuccinic acid, ↑ Cit, ↓ Arg; ↑ orotic acid (urine); enzyme studies: erythrocytes, fibroblasts

Argininaemia

Clinical: Relatively mild hyperammonaemia, rarely acute manifestation, progressive spasticity (equinus position of the feet), seizures and intellectual disability after the 2nd yr due to high arginine levels
Enzyme: Arginase; *ARG1* gene
Diagn.:   AA (plasma): ↑↑ Arg (*note*: may be normal in the neonate); ↑↑ orotic acid (urine); enzyme studies: erythrocytes
Therapy: Na-phenylbutyrate, Arg-restricted diet

HHH syndrome (hyperammonaemia, hyperornithinaemia, homocitrullinuria)

Clinical: Variable encephalopathy; clotting disorder with reduction of factors VII and X
Bioch.:   Disorder of ornithine transport between cytoplasm and mitochondrion
Diagn.:   AA (plasma): ↑↑ Orn (breakdown requires mitochondrial OAT, see *page 75*; normal values may be found in the neonate), n Arg, Cit; AA (urine): ↑ Orn, ↑ homocitrulline; enzyme studies: fibroblasts; *SLC25A15* gene
Therapy: Consider Orn supplementation (increases mitochondrial availability)

Citrullinaemia type II

Clinical: *Neonatal*: (transient) intrahepatic cholestasis, hepatomegaly (fatty liver), failure to thrive, hyperketotic hypoglycaemia
            Adult: recurrent encephalopathy, fatty liver, aversion to carbohydrate-rich food; pancreatitis, hepatoma
Bioch.:   Citrin deficiency; aspartate-glutamate carrier
Incidence: 1:17,000 in Japan; rare in Europe
Diagn.:   AA (plasma): ↑ Cit, Thr, Met, Tyr; *SLC25A13* gene
Therapy: Galactose-free diet, Na-benzoate, Na-phenylbutyrate, arginine; liver Tx

Other genetic defects of ammonia detoxification

- *N-Acetylglutamate synthase deficiency*: rare; usually severe disease (similar to CPS deficiency); efficient treatment with supplementation of carbamylglutamate (100–300 mg/kg/day); gene: *NAGS*
- *Hyperinsulinism-hyperammonaemia syndrome* (see *page 89*)
- *Lysinuric protein intolerance*: deficient transport of dibasic AA (see *page 76*)
- *Hypoprolinaemia* (see *page 75*; paradoxical fasting hyperammonaemia)
- *Glutamine synthetase deficiency* (see *page 77*; severe encephalopathy)

Biochemistry: Metabolism of branched-chain amino acids

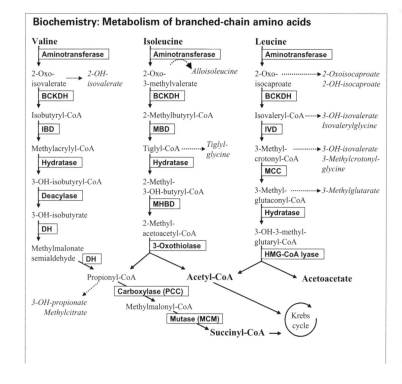

Branched-chain amino acids are metabolised predominantly in muscle and kidney. Together with succinyl-CoA they are important substrates of gluconeogenesis. Disorders affecting this pathway include maple syrup urine disease and the classical organic acidurias as well as various disorders of vitamin metabolism (cobalamin, biotin). Most disorders are diagnosed by the elevation of specific metabolites (e.g. methylcitric acid, 3-OH-isovaleric acid, methylmalonic acid) in urinary organic acid analysis.

Enzyme abbreviations: see description of individual disorders. DH = dehydrogenase.

Organic acidurias

Organic acidurias are disorders of intermediary metabolism with characteristic accumulation of carboxylic acids identified by GC/MS analysis of urine. Most patients present with systemic illness (classical organic acidurias) but it is now recognised that some have only cerebral abnormalities. The most common organic acidurias are caused by disorders involving the complex metabolism of branched-chain amino acids. The mitochondrial accumulation of CoA metabolites is an important difference between many organic acidurias and the aminoacidopathies.

Clinical: 1. *Neonatal form*: metabolic encephalopathy "intoxication type": lethargy, feeding problems, dehydration, truncal hypotonia/limb hypertonia, myoclonic jerks, neurovegetative dysregulation → cerebral oedema, coma, multi-organ failure; unusual odour

2. *Chronic intermittent form* (manifestation up to adulthood): recurrent episodes of ketoacidotic coma, lethargy and ataxia, focal neurological signs, stupor → coma, Reye syndrome

3. *Chronic progressive form*: failure to thrive, chronic vomiting, anorexia, osteoporosis, hypotonia, psychomotor retardation, recurrent infections (particularly candida)

Lab.:   Ketosis/ketoacidosis, ↑ lactate, ↑ NH_3, hypoglycaemia (or hyperglycaemia), neutropenia, thrombopenia, pancytopenia, ↓ calcium

Diagn.:   OA (urine): specific metabolites; carnitine status; acylcarnitines; enzyme studies; AA (plasma)

Therapy: (see *page 56*)

Acute: interrupt catabolic state with high-dose glucose infusion, counteract acidosis, stop protein intake, remove toxins, give carnitine, etc.

Long-term: diet – protein restriction; supplementation of unaffected amino acids (carefully check Ile, should be >25 μmol/l), minerals, vitamins, trace elements; carnitine

Compl.s: Demyelinisation, brain necrosis (basal ganglia), nephritis, pancreatitis, dermatoses → epidermolysis, osteoporosis, cardiomyopathy

"Cerebral" organic acidurias

Several organic acidurias present with (progressive) cerebral symptoms without basic laboratory abnormalities such as hypoglycaemia or metabolic/lactic acidosis. The diagnosis is made through the analysis of urinary organic acids, however, the specific metabolites are sometimes only slightly elevated and may be overlooked.

Clinical features include progressive ataxia, extrapyramidal signs, acute (epileptic) encephalopathy, macrocephaly, sometimes non-specific intellectual disability.

Neuroradiological findings include progressive demyelinisation (particularly spongiform encephalopathy), circumscribed brain atrophy, abnormalities in the basal ganglia, cerebellar hypoplasia/aplasia as well as symmetric and/or fluctuating abnormalities in the thalamus, hypothalamus, medulla and brain stem (DD: Leigh syndrome).

Glutaric aciduria type I (GA1)

Clinical: Macrocephaly, fronto-temporal atrophy; acute encephalopathic crisis (usually age 6–18 mths) with destruction of the striatum, subsequently severe dystonic-dyskinetic movement disorder; leukoencephalopathy in adulthood

Enzyme: Glutaryl-CoA dehydrogenase in Lys/Trp metabolism (see *page 72*); *GCDH* gene

Diagn.:   OA (urine): ↑ glutaric acid, 3-OH-glutaric acid (diagnostic); ↓ carnitine; acylcarnitines: ↑ glutarylcarnitine; enzyme studies (leukocytes); *note*: metabolic abnormalities may be fluctuating and inconsistent

DD: Mitochondrial disorders; GA type II = multiple acyl-CoA dehydrogenase deficiency (*page 94*); GA type III = probably non-disease caused by mutations in the C7orf10 gene coding for a possible CoA transferase protein

Therapy: Strict adherence to emergency protocol in infancy and early childhood; carnitine 100 mg/kg/day, diet (Lys- and Trp-restricted, beware of Trp deficiency!)

Propionic aciduria (PA)

Enzyme: Propionyl-CoA carboxylase; *PCCA* and *PCCB* genes

Bioch.:   Biotin-dependent enzyme (but no biotin-responsive patient reported); propionyl-CoA inhibits enzymes of the Krebs cycle, the urea cycle and other pathways

Diagn.:   OA (urine): ↑ 3-OH-propionic and methylcitric acids, ↑ C_5 and C_6 ketones; ↓ carnitine; acylcarnitines: ↑ propionylcarnitine; AA (plasma): ↑ Gly, Ala

DD: Disorders of biotin metabolism

Therapy: Diet (↓ Ile, Val, Met, Thr; corresponding to valine tolerance); L-carnitine (50–)100 mg/kg/day; consider metronidazole (10–20 mg/kg) and/or colistin for 10 days/mth (↓ enteral propionic acid and NH_3)

Compl.s: Intellectual disability, extrapyramidal movement disorder, osteoporosis, pancreatitis, cardiomyopathy

Methylmalonic aciduria (MMA)

Elevation of methylmalonic acid is found in a large number of inherited and non-genetic disorders such as mitochondrial disorders or nutritive cobalamin (cbl, vit. B_{12}) deficiency. The most common monogenic cause of high methylmalonic acid excretion is methylmalonyl-CoA mutase (MCM) deficiency. Secondary MCM deficiency may also be caused by deficient biosynthesis of its cofactor cobalamin (see *page 156*).

Enzyme: Methylmalonyl-CoA mutase (MCM); *MUT* gene

Variants: Mut⁻: residual function, cbl-responsiveness; Mut⁰: no residual function

Diagn.:   OA (urine): ↑ methylmalonic, 3-OH-propionic and methylcitric acids; ↓ carnitine; acylcarnitines; AA (plasma): ↑ Gly, Ala

DD: Disorders of vit. B_{12} (cobalamin) metabolism, vit. B_{12} deficiency

Therapy: Trial of vit. B_{12} (hydroxocobalamin): acute 2 mg/day for one week i.v.; work-up in a stable metabolic state: 1 mg/day s.c. for three days; careful biochemical monitoring (urinary MMA should fall by >50%); otherwise like propionic aciduria

Compl.s: Intellectual disability, extrapyramidal movement disorders; osteoporosis; *progressive renal failure* (*note*: creatinine is unreliable for the assessment of renal function [low protein diet, reduced muscle mass] – determine GFR)

Mildly elevated urinary methylmalonic acid (miscellaneous disorders)

- *Methylmalonyl-CoA epimerase deficiency* (*MCEE* gene): clinical consequences uncertain
- *Succinate-CoA ligase* (*SUCL*) *enzyme complex deficiency*: MMA is likely to constitute a marker of the disease rather than to be responsible for the phenotype.
  - *SUCLA2* mutations: encephalomyopathy and mtDNA depletion
  - *SUCLG1*: fatal infantile lactic acidosis of neonatal onset with mtDNA depletion

Isovaleric aciduria (IVA)

Enzyme:	Isovaleryl-CoA dehydrogenase; *IVD* gene
Bioch.:	FAD-dependent enzyme (→ electron-transfer flavoprotein; see *page 99*)
Diagn.:	OA (urine): ↑↑ isovalerylglycine, 3-OH-isovaleric acid; ↓ carnitine; acylcarnitines: ↑ isovalerylcarnitine
Therapy:	L-Carnitine (50–)100 mg/kg/day ± glycine 150–250 mg/kg/day; diet (Leu-restricted or low protein)
Progn.:	Good if diagnosis is not delayed and strict therapy is maintained

3-Methylglutaconic acidurias (MGAs)

Heterogeneous group of disorders characterised by excretion of 3-methylglutaconic acid. Type I is an inborn error of leucine catabolism; the other types all affect mitochondrial function through different pathomechanisms. Treatment is largely symptomatic.

Type IV:	*Unclassified* (largest group): variable clinical symptoms, intellectual disability, neurological abnormalities
Type I:	*3-Methylglutaconyl-CoA hydratase deficiency*: slowly progressive leukoencephalopathy presenting in adulthood, incidental finding in childhood (*AUH* gene)
Type II:	*Barth syndrome*: X-linked (cardio)myopathy, growth retardation, neutropenia; deficiency of tafazzin (mitochondrial membrane protein) affecting phospholipid metabolism (*TAZ* gene)
Type III:	*Costeff syndrome*: optic atrophy, extrapyramidal signs, spasticity; deficiency of a mitochondrial membrane protein (*OPA3* gene)
Type V:	*DCMA syndrome*: dilated cardiomyopathy with conduction defects and non-progressive cerebellar ataxia (*DNAJC19* gene)
Other:	*Hypertrophic cardiomyopathy*, lactic acidosis: *TMEM70* mutations
	Encephalomyopathy, neurodegenerative symptoms: *SUCLA2* mutations
	Hepatocerebral phenotype: *POLG1* mutations (mtDNA-depletion; *page 106*)
	Myopathy, central core disease: *RYR1* mutations

3-Methylcrotonylglycinuria

Clinical:	Common benign condition; pathogenic relevance unproven
Enzyme:	3-Methylcrotonyl-CoA carboxylase; *MCCC1 and MCCC2* genes
Bioch.:	Biotin-dependent enzyme
Diagn.:	OA (urine): ↑ 3-OH-isovaleric acid, 3-methylcrotonylglycine; ↓ carnitine
DD:	Disorders of biotin metabolism
Therapy:	Not usually necessary; consider L-carnitine if carnitine very low

D-2-hydroxyglutaric aciduria

Clinical: Variable; developmental delay, epilepsy, hypotonia, cardiomyopathy, dysmorphic features; sometimes asymptomatic; data on differences between type I and II not yet available

Type I: D-2-hydroxyglutarate dehydrogenase deficiency; *D2HGDH* gene

Type II: Heterozygous gain of function mutations (p.R140Q, p.R140G) in the mitochondrial isocitrate dehydrogenase gene (*IDH2*)

Diagn.:   OA (urine, CSF): ↑ 2-hydroxyglutaric acid, enantiomer analysis: D-Form

Therapy: Symptomatic

L-2-hydroxyglutaric aciduria

Clinical: Psychomotor retardation, epilepsy, cerebellar ataxia, macrocephaly; often slowly progressive; peripheral leukodystrophy (U-fibres), symmetric high signal (T2w) of dentate nucleus and pallidum

Enzyme: L-2-Hydroxyglutarate dehydrogenase; *L2HGDH* gene

Diagn.:   OA (urine, CSF): ↑ 2-hydroxyglutaric acid, enantiomer analysis: L-Form; AA (CSF): ↑ lysine

Therapy: Satisfactory control of seizures with anti-epileptic medication (control of 'minor' fits can be difficult)

Ethylmalonic aciduria

Ethylmalonic acid can be derived from either the carboxylation of butyryl-CoA in fatty acid oxidation or from the R-pathway of isoleucine metabolism.

Disease	Additional features	Page
SCAD deficiency	Probably non-disease; ↑ butyrylcarnitine, -glycine	94
Multiple acyl-CoA dehydrogenase deficiency	Metabolic acidosis, hypoglycaemia, hypotonia, dysmorphic features, malodour; various other organic acids (glutaric, adipic, lactic acids, etc.)	94
Jamaican vomiting sickness	Hypoglycin poisoning (ingestion of unripe ackee fruit)	

Ethylmalonic encephalopathy

Clinical: Neurodevelopmental regression, pyramidal and extrapyramidal tract signs, seizures, petechiae, orthostatic acrocyanosis, chronic diarrhoea; CNS malformations; multiple lesions on MRI; lethal in infancy or early childhood

Protein: Mitochondrial matrix protein encoded by *ETHE1* gene

Diagn.:   Lactic acidaemia; acylcarnitines: ↑ C_4, C_5; OA (urine): ↑ ethylmalonic acid, methylsuccinic acid, C_4–C_6 acylglycines; COX deficiency in muscle

Therapy: Symptomatic

2-Methyl-3-hydroxybutyric aciduria

Clinical: *Males*: progressive neurodegeneration, loss of skills, choreoathetosis, epilepsy, blindness; mild acidosis in catabolic states, cardiomyopathy
Females may have non-progressive intellectual disability.

Protein: 2-Methyl-3-hydroxybutyryl-CoA dehydrogenase (MHBD) = 17β-hydroxysteroid dehydrogenase type 10 (HSD10); clinical symptoms unrelated to enzyme function

Genetics: X-chromosomal; *HSD17B10* gene

Diagn.: OA (urine): ↑ 2-Methyl-3-hydroxybutyrate, tiglylglycine, normal 2-methylacetoacetate; acylcarnitines usually normal; enzyme studies

Other organic acidurias

- *Multiple acyl-CoA dehydrogenase deficiency* (FAD-dependent enzymes) (see *page 94*)
- *Multiple carboxylase deficiency* (biotin-dependent enzymes) (see *page 159*)
- *HMG-CoA lyase deficiency* (see *page 94*)
- *3-Oxothiolase deficiency* (see *page 95*)

Other cerebral organic acidurias

- *4-Hydroxybutyric aciduria*: succinic semialdehyde dehydrogenase deficiency (see *page 154*)
- *Malonic aciduria* (malonyl-CoA decarboxylase deficiency; *MLYCD* gene): relatively mild clinical features; developmental retardation, epilepsy, recurrent vomiting; therapy: carnitine supplementation, low-fat high-carbohydrate diet (experimental)
- *Canavan disease*: progressive psychomotor retardation, progressive epileptic encephalopathy, macrocephaly, leukodystrophy (particularly subcortical U-fibres), optic atrophy; enzyme: Aspartoacylase; diagn.: OA (urine): ↑ N-acetylaspartic acid; acylcarnitines normal; enzyme studies; gene: *ASPA*; therapy: symptomatic
- *See also*: mitochondrial disorders (*page 96*)

Organic acidurias of doubtful clinical relevance

- *Isobutyric aciduria*: incidental finding in newborn screening (isobutyryl-CoA dehydrogenase [IBD] deficiency, valine metabolism, *ACAD8* gene)
- *3-Hydroxyisobutyric aciduria*: possibly incidental finding; gene unknown
- *Methylmalonate semialdehyde dehydrogenase deficiency*: various OA abnormalities, poorly characterised clinical picture and genetic basis
- *2-Methylbutyric aciduria*: incidental finding in newborn screening (2-methylbutyryl-CoA dehydrogenase [MBD] deficiency, isoleucine metabolism, *ACADSB* gene)

Disorders of the metabolism of branched-chain amino acids not classified as organic aciduria

Biochemistry: see *page 60*

Maple syrup urine disease (MSUD)

The clinical picture of maple syrup urine disease, as in other aminoacidopathies, is caused by the specific action of toxic metabolites (particularly 2-oxoisocaproic acid). In contrast to the classical organic acidurias there is no accumulation of CoA metabolites (no characteristic acylcarnitines), and acidosis or hyperammonaemia are not major features of the disease.

Clinical: *Severe form*: progressive encephalopathy from the 3rd–5th days of life: lethargy, feeding problems, somnolence, cerebral oedema, coma
             Mild form: psychomotor retardation, fluctuating/progressive neurological disease, recurrent ketoacidotic decompensation (DD: ketonaemic vomiting)
             Urine odour may be highly characteristic (maple syrup-like)

Enzyme: Branched-chain α-oxoacid dehydrogenase (BCKDH) complex = multi-enzyme complex similar to pyruvate dehydrogenase (PDH) complex; Proteins/genes: $E_{1\alpha}$/*BCKDHA*, $E_{1\beta}$/*BCKDHB*, E_2/*DBT*, E_3/*DLD*

Incidence: In Europe approx. 1:200,000

Diagn.:   AA (plasma): ↑ Val, ↑↑ Leu, Ile, alloisoleucine (diagnostic)
             OA (urine): ↑ branched-chain oxo- and hydroxyacids, e.g. 2-OH-isovaleric acid, 2-oxo-isocaproic acid E_3 deficiency: combined deficiency of several mitochondrial dehydrogenases (see PDH deficiency; *page 97*)

Therapy: *Acute*: glucose + insulin i.v.; enhance protein anabolism (avoid secondary deficiency of Ile and Val by early supplementation); exchange transfusion/dialysis not usually required
             Long-term: diet (monitor plasma Leu, Val, Ile); consider trial of thiamine for 3 wks (10 mg/kg/day; see also *page 161*)
             Range of optimal therapy: Leu 100–250 µmol/l
                                          Ile 50–150 µmol/l
                                          Val 150–250 µmol/l

Progn.:   Satisfactory with prompt (before the 5th day of life) and strict therapy

Other disorders involving branched-chain amino acids

* *Hyperleucine-isoleucinaemia* and *hypervalinaemia*: rare conditions of uncertain relevance, may be caused by branched-chain aminotransferase deficiency
* *3-Hydroxyisobutyryl-CoA hydrolyse* (*deacylase*) deficiency (valine metabolism): failure to thrive, neurological regression in infancy, episodes of ketoacidosis, Leigh-like MRI changes; diagn.: ↓ OH-C_4-carnitine, ↑ cysteine and cysteamine conjugates of methacrylic acid (urine); *HIBCH* gene

For organic acidurias involving branched-chain amino acid metabolism see *page 61*.

Disorders of phenylalanine and tyrosine metabolism

Biochemistry

Phenylalanine and tyrosine metabolism takes place in the cytosol. A deficiency of the enzyme *phenylalanine hydroxylase* (PAH) or the cofactor tetrahydrobiopterin (BH_4) causes the accumulation of phenylalanine which is transaminated to phenylpyruvate. The cleavage of the phenolic ring is only possible by dioxygenation of homogentisate.

A deficiency of the enzyme *fumarylacetoacetase* causes accumulation of fumarylacetoacetate and succinylacetoacetate and -acetone. These highly toxic substances inhibit several enzymes incl. 4-OH-phenylpyruvate dioxygenase and aminolaevulinate dehydratase and are carcinogenic (alkylation of DNA).

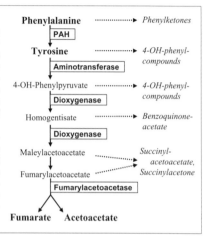

Phenylketonuria (PKU)

PKU was one of the first neurogenetic disorders identified (Følling 1934), the first successfully treated inborn error of metabolism (diet: Bickel 1953) and the disorder that was instrumental for the introduction of neonatal population screening (dried blood spots: Guthrie 1963).

Clinical: Untreated: severe brain damage with intellectual disability, seizures, spasticity

Variants: *PKU*: requires diet (differences in disease severity/Phe tolerance: severe PKU = homozygous null mutation, mild PKU = at least one hypomorphic/residual function mutation)

MHP: mild hyperphenylalaninaemia, does not require diet therapy (Phe <600 μmol/l in Germany, <400 μmol/l in the UK, <420 μmol/l in the USA)

"*BH_4-sensitive PKU*": reduction of Phe levels after BH_4 supplementation in many patients with mild PKU (stabilisation/activation of mutant protein)

Enzyme: Phenylalanine hydroxylase; *PAH* gene

Genetics: >600 mutations in the *PAH* gene, varying residual activities (see *PAH* mutation database: www.pahdb.mcgill.ca)

Incidence: In Europe up to 1:4,400 (Ireland), average ~1:8,000

Diagn.: Newborn screening (filter paper card), AA (plasma): ↑ Phe, n–↓ Tyr; mutation analysis may allow prediction of severity and BH_4 sensitivity

DD: BH_4 cofactor deficiency (see *page 153*)

Therapy: Phe-restricted diet, supplementation of essential amino acids + trace elements (exact recommendations differ between countries; see below for the German recommendations); BH_4 supplementation in mild PKU (not all patients)

Progn.: Normal development and intelligence with immediate and efficient treatment

Maternal PKU

Fetopathy in pregnant mothers with PKU (Phe >360 μmol/l); strict diet treatment must be started before conception and maintained throughout pregnancy!

German recommendations for PKU treatment

Goal:	1ˢᵗ–10ᵗʰ yr:	Phe values 40–240 μmol/l (0.7–4 mg/dl)
	11ᵗʰ–16ᵗʰ yr:	Phe values 40–900 μmol/l (0.7–15 mg/dl)
	After 16 yrs:	Phe values < 1,200 μmol/l (< 20 mg/dl)
	During pregnancy:	Phe values 120–360 μmol/l (2–6 mg/dl)
Follow-up:	1ˢᵗ yr:	Lab every 1–2 wks, clinical every 3 mths
	2ⁿᵈ–10ᵗʰ yr:	Lab every 2–4 wks, clinical every 3–6 mths
	11ᵗʰ–16ᵗʰ yr:	Lab every 4 wks, clinical every 6 mths
	After 16 yrs:	Lab every 2–3 mths, clinical every 6–12 mths

Tyrosinaemia type I

Clinical:	*Acute (neonate/infant)*: severe liver failure, vomiting, bleeding, septicaemia, hypoglycaemia, renal tubulopathy (Fanconi syndrome)
	Chronic: hepatomegaly, cirrhosis, growth retardation, rickets, haematoma, tubulopathy, neuropathy, neurological crises (due to porphyrins)
Enzyme:	Fumarylacetoacetase; *FAH* gene
Diagn.:	OA (urine): (n–) ↑ Succinylacetone (diagnostic), ↑ 4-OH-phenyl derivatives; AA (plasma): (n–)↑ Tyr, ↑ Met (!); (n–)↑ α-fetoprotein (serum); porphyrins (urine): ↑ δ-aminolaevulinic acid; aminolaevulinate dehydratase activity (possible in DBS)
DD:	Liver disorders, in particular "neonatal hepatitis", respiratory chain defects, galactosaemia, fructose intolerance, bile acid synthesis disorders
Therapy:	Nitisinone (NTBC) 1(–2) mg/kg in 2 doses (inhibitor of 4-OH-phenylpyruvate dioxygenase, blocks the accumulation of toxic metabolites; beware of ↑Tyr); Phe- + Tyr-restricted diet; liver transplantation probably not longer needed in most patients
Progn.:	With nitisinone good (long-term prognosis still unclear)
Compl.s:	Hepatocellular carcinoma (watch AFP), renal failure

Tyrosinaemia type II

Clinical:	Painful corneal lesions (lacrimation, photophobia, scars), hyperkeratosis (soles, palms), mild intellectual disability
Enzyme:	Cytosolic tyrosine aminotransferase; *TAT* gene
Diagn.:	AA (plasma): ↑↑ Tyr, ↑ Phe; OA (urine): 4-OH-phenylpyruvate, -lactate, -acetate
Therapy:	Phe- and Tyr-restricted diet

Alkaptonuria

Clinical:	Black/brown/red urine discolouration at alkaline pH; arthritis, cardiac valve disease
Enzyme:	Homogentisate dioxygenase; *HGD* gene
Diagn.:	OA (urine): ↑↑ homogentisic acid
Therapy:	Low-protein diet, possibly NTBC (study)

Other disorders of tyrosine metabolism

- Tyrosinaemia type III: 4-Hydroxyphenylpyruvate dioxygenase deficiency, *HPD* gene; uncertain clinical relevance, no skin lesions; a Phe and Tyr-restricted diet is recommended
- Hawkinsinuria: unknown enzyme; doubtful clinical relevance; failure to thrive, acidosis

Disorders of the metabolism of sulphur amino acids

Biochemistry (incl. folic acid cycle/cytosolic methyl group transfer)

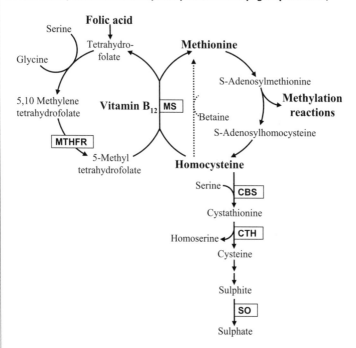

S-Adenosylmethionine (SAM), is the most important methyl group donor in cellular metabolism. Remethylation of homocysteine to methionine is catalysed mainly by the cobalamin-(vit. B_{12}-)dependent methionine synthase (MS) or alternatively betaine-homocysteine methyltransferase (methyl group donor betaine). The methyl group is transferred onto cob(I) alamin (cbl^I) from 5,10-methylenetetrahydrofolate which is regenerated in the folate cycle. The breakdown of homocysteine to cysteine is catalysed by the vit. B_6-dependent enzymes cystathionine beta-synthase (CBS) und cystathionine gamma-lyase (CTH). Cysteine is further catabolised via cysteine sulphinate (precursor of the amino acid taurine, a component of the bile acids) to sulphite which is oxidised to sulphate by the molybdenum-containing enzyme sulphite oxidase (SO) and excreted in the urine.

Methionine and homocysteine play a central role in cytosolic methyl group transfer required for a range of functions incl. the synthesis of creatine, choline and adrenaline as well as DNA methylation. Disorders of the cytosolic methyl group transfer may also be due to primary disorders of cobalamin (vit. B$_{12}$) or folate metabolism (see *pages 156, 157*); they frequently cause severe neurological disorders; symptoms may also be related to vascular complications of elevated homocysteine.

Homocysteine (Hcy) and cysteine (Cys) are usually found as disulphides (homocystine and cystine) in the extracellular space. Mild elevations of Hcy in plasma (centrifuge immediately, analysis see *page 33*) can only be detected through a specific method (e.g. HPLC). Classical homocystinuria, however, may also be recognised by a positive nitroprusside test (Brand reaction, see *page 31*) in the urine. Cystinosis (*page 141*) and cystinuria (*page 76*) are caused by lysosomal and renal transport defects.

Isolated hypermethioninaemia

Clinical: Often asymptomatic, cabbage-like odour, intellectual disability, neurological disease, demyelination

Enzyme: Methionine adenosyltransferase I/III; *MAT1A* gene

Diagn.:   ↑↑ Met

Therapy: In symptomatic patients, Met-restricted diet and/or SAM administration

DD: *Glycine N-methyltransferase deficiency* (*GNMT* gene): ↑↑ Met, SAM; ↓ S-adenosylhomcysteine; may be a coincidental finding

S-Adenosylhomocysteine hydrolase deficiency

Clinical: Progressive intellectual disability, neurological disease, hypomyelination and white matter atrophy

Diagn.:   ↑ Met; ↑↑ SAM; S-adenosylhomcysteine; ↑ CK; gene: *AHCY*

Therapy: Met-restricted diet

Methionine synthase deficiency (cblG disease)

Clinical: Megaloblastic anaemia, progressive intellectual disability, neurological disease, psychiatric disturbance

Diagn.:   ↑ Hcy (> 150 μmol/l); AA (plasma): n–↓ Met; OA (urine): ↑ methylmalonic acid (cobalamin defects); nitroprusside test positive; gene: *MTR*

Therapy: HO-cobalamin (1 mg/day–week i.m., dose depends on defect); consider betaine (75 mg/kg/day) and folic acid 5–10 mg/day

DD: *Methionine synthase reductase deficiency:* cblE disease, *MTRR* gene; activation/regeneration of catalytically inert cbl^{II} (formed every 200–1,000 MS catalytic cycles) to cbl^{I}

Mild hyperhomocysteinaemia

Clinical: Risk factor (particularly in conjunction with folate deficiency) for premature vascular disease in the 3rd and 4th decade (infarctions, thromboembolism – not relevant in child-hood); ↑ Risk for neural tube defects in maternal hyperhomocysteinaemia

Causes: • Endogenous and exogenous disorders of folic acid or homocysteine metabolism, es-pecially folate deficiency + homozygosity for MTHFR polymorphism p.A222V (c.665C>T; traditional: 677C>T oder C677T homozygous in up to 5% of Europeans)
• Vit. B_{12} deficiency

Diagn.: ↑ tHcy (plasma) > 15 (up to 30–40) μmol/l

Therapy: Folic acid 5 mg/day, sometimes vit. B_6 (pyridoxine) 100 mg/day

Classical homocystinuria

Clinical: Marfan-like appearance, epilepsy, intellectual disability, progressive myopia (early symptom), lens dislocation, osteoporosis, thromboembolism

Manif.: Progressive disease, usually starting at school age

Enzyme: Cystathionine beta-synthase (*CBS* gene)

Bioch.: Varying severity of enzyme deficiency, accumulation of homocysteine → collagen dis-order

Diagn.: AA (plasma): ↑ Met, ↑↑ Hcy (>150 μmol/l), ↓ Cys; nitroprusside test positive

DD: Disorders of methionine synthesis; cobalamin defects

Therapy: Pyridoxine 50–100 mg/day (+ folic acid 10 mg/day); if this has no effect: Met-restricted diet, betaine 100 mg/kg/day (if necessary up to 3 × 3 g/day), hydroxocobalamin (1 mg/day orally, from 5 yrs of age), vit. C (100 mg/day)
Goal: Hcy (plasma) < 30 μmol/l (one may be doing well at 60 μmol/l)

Sulphite oxidase deficiency and molybdenum cofactor deficiency

Molybdenum cofactor (MoCo) consists of molybdenum bound to a modified pterin. It is required for four enzymes incl. xanthine oxidoreductase (see *page 114*) and sulfite oxidase (*SUOX* gene). MoCo biosynthesis involves three proteins encoded by the genes *MOCS1*, *MOCS2* and *GEPH*. Clinical symptoms are identical in MoCo deficiency and isolated sulphite oxidase deficiency (less common).

Clinical: Infantile epileptic encephalopathy; progressive psychomotor retardation, severe mi-crocephaly; later: lens dislocation

Diagn.: Sulphite test (*fresh* urine) positive; AA (plasma): ↑ taurine, ↑ sulphocysteine, ↓ Cys, ↓ Hcy; enzyme studies
MoCo deficiency: ↓↓ uric acid (serum), ↑↑ (hypo)xanthine (purines in urine); muta-tions: *MOCS1*>*MOCS2*; only one patient with *GEPH* mutation

Therapy: Substitution of cPMP in MoCo deficiency type A (*MOCS1* mutations); no specific therapy for type B (*MOCS2*) or isolated sulphite oxidase deficiency

Other disorders involving sulphur-amino acids

• Cystathioninuria (cystathionine gamma-lyase deficiency, *CTH* gene) is generally considered to be a benign condition without pathogenetic relevance.

Disorders of histidine, tryptophan and lysine metabolism

Biochemistry

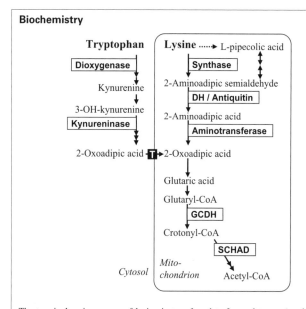

The terminal amino group of lysine is transferred to 2-oxoglutarate (producing glutamate and involving the intermediary saccharopine) in a two-step reaction catalysed by 2-aminoadipic semialdehyde synthase (AASS). An alternative pathway involving the intermediate L-pipecolic acid may be predominant in the brain. 2-Aminoadipic semialdehyde is dehydrogenated to 2-aminoadipic acid and transaminated to 2-oxoadipic acid. Tryptophan is metabolised in a complex cytosolic pathway to kynurenine and subsequently also 2-oxoadipic acid. 2-Oxoadipic acid is transported into the mitochondrion and metabolised to glutaryl-CoA and crotonyl-CoA in two consecutive oxidative decarboxylation steps (the first one involves the intermediary glutaric acid). Histidine is deaminated by histidase to urocanate and subsequently converted by urocanase and a hydrolase to N-formimino-L-glutamate. The formimino group is transferred onto tetrahydrofolate, giving rise to 5,10-methenyltetrahydrofolate which is used in the folate cycle.

Glutaric aciduria type I
See *page 62*

Histidinaemia
Clinical: Incidental finding, asymptomatic
Enzyme: Histidase/histidine ammonialyase; *HAL* gene
Diagn.:   AA (plasma): ↑ His; AA (urine): ↑ His; ↑ imidazolepyruvic acid (urine)
Therapy: None required

Tryptophanaemia

Clinical: Incidental finding, asymptomatic; occasional symptoms of nicotinic acid deficiency (as in Hartnup disease, see *page 76*)

Enzyme: Tryptophan-2,3-dioxygenase?

Incidence: Approx. 1:10,000

Diagn.:   AA (plasma): ↑ Trp (400–800 µmol/l)

Therapy: Nicotinamide (50–300 mg/day)

Other disorders of histidine, lysine and tryptophan metabolism

- *Urocanic aciduria*: probably asymptomatic; deficient urocanase (*UROC1* gene)
- *Formiminotransferase deficiency*: mostly asymptomatic; ↑ formiminoglutamic acid (urine); *FTCD* gene. Treatment with folinic acid (15 mg/day) has been tried in symptomatic patients with folate deficiency.
- *Hyperlysinaemia*: rare, deficiency of 2-aminoadipic semialdehyde synthase (*AASS* gene); uncertain clinical relevance
- 2-aminoadipic semialdehyde dehydrogenase (antiquitin) deficiency: see pyridoxine-responsive epilepsy; *page 160* (*ALDH7A1* gene)
- *2-Aminoadipic aciduria*: rare, uncertain molecular basis, uncertain relevance; urinary oxoadipic acid may be cytosolic in origin
- *Hydroxykynureninuria*: rare, ? deficiency of kynureninase; treatment: nicotinamide
- *Hydroxylysinuria*: last reported in the 1970s

Disorders of serine, glycine and glycerate metabolism

Biochemistry

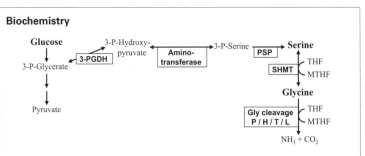

Serine is formed from 3-phosphoglycerate (glycolysis) and is used for the synthesis of cysteine, purines, thymine and other metabolites. It can deaminated to pyruvate via pyridoxal phosphate-(PALP-)dependent serine dehydratase (which also converts threonine to 2-oxobutyrate + NH_4^+) and thus may serve as a substrate of gluconeogenesis. Serine is reversibly converted to glycine by serine hydroxymethyltransferase (SHMT, also PALP-dependent) which employs tetrahydrofolate (THF) as a methyl group acceptor; this reaction represents one step in the folate cycle (*page 69*). Gly also serves as the main inhibitory neurotransmitter. It is broken down by the mitochondrial glycine cleavage system, an enzyme complex consisting of four proteins (P, H, T, L) and resembling the pyruvate dehydrogenase complex.

Serine deficiency disorders

Disorders of serine synthesis have only been diagnosed in few children.
* *3-Phosphoglycerate dehydrogenase deficiency*: congenital microcephaly; psychomotor retardation, epilepsy, spastic tetraparesis; attenuated form with moderate intellectual disability; *PGDH* gene
* *3-Phosphoserine aminotransferase deficiency*: one patient with intellectual disability, postnatal microcephaly; sibling asymptomatic on serine treatment; *PSAT* gene
* *3-Phosphoserine phosphatase deficiency*: one boy with Williams syndrome (no epilepsy, normal glycine); *PSPH* gene

Diagn.: AA (CSF + plasma, fasting!): ↓ Ser; n–↓ Gly; ↓ 5-methyltetrahydrofolate in CSF; enzyme studies: fibroblasts

Therapy: L-serine 200–600 mg/kg/day until normalisation of L-serine; if seizures persist add glycine up to 200 mg/kg/day

Non-ketotic hyperglycinaemia

Clinical: Severe epileptic encephalopathy, hypotonia, progressive neurological symptoms; neonatal onset, variants with late onset or transient disease course

Enzyme: Glycine cleavage system

Diagn.: AA (plasma, CSF): ↑ Gly, Gly-ratio CSF/plasma >0.08 (normal <0.02); *caution*: borderline elevations can be caused by valproate treatment; enzyme studies: lymphocytes, liver; mutations: *GLDC* (P protein; >50% of families), *AMT* (T protein), *GCSH* (H protein; rare)
Variant enzyme defects have been shown to result in less severe variable phenotypes and CSF/plasma ratios >0.02 and <0.08.

DD: *Hyperglycinaemia (with ketosis)*: organic acidurias (inhibition of hepatic glycine cleavage system by pathological metabolites); prolonged fasting

Therapy: Experimental dextromethorphan (5–20 mg/kg/day), Na-benzoate (250–750 mg/kg/day, aiming to normalise plasma glycine levels with plasma benzoate levels below 2,000 μM); folinic acid (15 mg/day)

Progn.: Poor

Other disorders of serine, glycine and glycerate metabolism

* *Sarcosinaemia:* sarcosine dehydrogenase deficiency (sarcosine is produced in the breakdown of choline via betaine to glycine); probably incidental finding; ↑ sarcosine identified by AA analysis (plasma, urine)
* *D-glyceric aciduria:* rare, may be incidental; ↑ glyceric acid identified by OA analysis (urine); *GLYCTK* gene

Disorders of ornithine, proline and hydroxyproline metabolism

Biochemistry

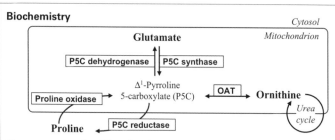

The concentration of ornithine, the primary carrier molecule of the urea cycle (see *page 57*), is regulated by *ornithine aminotransferase* (OAT). The reversible reaction catalysed by this enzyme allows ornithine synthesis at times of high arginine requirements, e.g. in the first months of life, whilst later in life it is required for removal of dietary arginine. The intermediary product, Δ^1-pyrroline-5-carboxylate (P5C), may be synthesised from glutamate and is also the precursor of proline.

Gyrate atrophy of retina and choroidea

Clinical: Myopia (childhood), impaired night vision → blindness (age 40–55 yrs); fundoscopy: Retinopathy (gyrate atrophy, increasing from the periphery)
Enzyme: Ornithine aminotransferase (*OAT* gene)
Bioch.: Disorder of ornithine removal (toxic on retinal cells)
Diagn.: NH_3 normal (except occasionally in neonates); AA (plasma): ↑ Orn; ↓ creatinine
DD: Urea cycle defects (HHH syndrome)
Therapy: Pyridoxine 40–200–600 mg/day; arginine-restricted diet; consider creatine monophosphate (up to 2 g/kg/day); Arg in hyperammonaemic neonates

Hyperprolinaemia

Type I: Proline oxidase deficiency; incidental finding, mostly asymptomatic, associated with schizophrenia; *PRODH* gene
Type II: Δ^1-Pyrroline-5-carboxylate (P5C) dehydrogenase deficiency; associated with epilepsy, intellectual disability; may be asymptomatic; secondary deficiency of PLP (vit. B_6), see *page 159*; *ALDH4A1* gene

Diagn.: AA (plasma): ↑ ↑ Pro; AA (urine): ↑ Pro, OH-Pro, Gly; *type II*: ↑ P5C (plasma, urine)
Therapy: Epilepsy may respond to pyridoxine 50 mg orally per day

Other disorders of proline and hydroxyproline metabolism

- *Hypoprolinaemia* (Δ^1-pyrroline-5-carboxylate (P5C) synthase deficiency): *cataract*; *joint* hypermobility; progressive intellectual disability; hyperammonaemia; AA (plasma): ↓ Pro; ↓ Orn; ↓ Arg; ↓ Cit; P5CS gene
- *Δ^1-Pyrroline-5-carboxylate (P5C) reductase deficiency:* cutis laxa, wrinkly skin, osteopenia, progeroid appearance; no metabolic abnormalities reported; *PYCR1* gene
- *Hydroxyprolinaemia* (hydroxy-L-proline oxidase deficiency): probably non-disease; AA (plasma): ↑ hydroxyproline, ↑ XLE (newborn screening for MSUD, see *page 50*)

Disorders of amino acid transport

Several specific transport systems ensure virtually complete (re)absorption of amino acids in the gut and kidneys. The calculation of renal tubular re-absorption shows values ≥ 95–99% for most amino acids. Genetic defects of these transport systems are sometimes asymptomatic and are detected only through elevation of the respective amino acids in urine with normal (or low) values in plasma.

Lysinuric protein intolerance

Clinical: Failure to thrive, diarrhoea, interstitional pneumonia, osteoporosis, renal failure, haemolysis, hyperammonaemia with progressive encephalopathy – prevalent in Finland

Bioch.:   (Re)absorption defect of the dibasic amino acids (Lys, Arg, Orn) → interruption of the urea cycle; lysine deficiency; *SLC7A7* gene

Diagn.:   ↑ NH$_3$, LDH, ferritin; AA (urine): ↑ Arg, Lys, Orn; AA (plasma): n–↓ Arg, Lys, Orn, n–↑ citrulline; enzyme studies: liver

Therapy: Citrulline substitution, protein restriction (does not correct Lys deficiency)

Cystinuria

Clinical: Nephrolithiasis (cystine crystallises above 1,250 μmol/l at pH 7.5)

Bioch.:   Re-absorption defect of Lys, Arg, Orn and Cys

Type A: *SLC3A1* mutations (heterozygotes have normal urinary AA = type I)

Type B: *SLC7A9* mutations (most heterozygotes ↑ urine Cys, Lys = type II/III)

Diagn.:   Nitroprusside test positive; AA (urine): ↑↑ Cys, ↑ Arg, Lys, Orn; AA (plasma): normal

Therapy: High fluid intake, also at night (> 5 l/day); alkalinisation of the urine; in selected cases try penicillamine 1–2 g/day; consider mercaptopropionylglycine or captopril

Hartnup disease

Clinical: Often asymptomatic; sometimes photodermatitis, cerebellar ataxia

Bioch.:   Reabsorption defect of the neutral amino acids (Ala, Ser, Thr, Val, Leu, Ile, Phe, Tyr, Trp, His, Gln, Asn); pathogenetically relevant: tryptophan deficiency → nicotinic acid and serotonin deficiency; *SLC6A19* gene

Diagn.:   AA (urine): ↑ neutral amino acids; AA (plasma): n–↓ neutral amino acids

DD: Fanconi syndrome: ↑ all AA incl. Pro (!), Gly, Arg, Lys, Orn

Therapy: Nicotinamide 50–300 mg/day; sun protection

Iminoglycinuria

Clinical: Incidental finding, asymptomatic

Bioch.:   Reabsorption defect of imino acids (Pro, hydroxyproline) and Gly

Diagn.:   AA (urine): ↑ Pro, OH-Pro, Gly

DD: Hyperprolinaemia, hydroxyprolinaemia (AA plasma!), Fanconi syndrome

Other disorders of amino acid metabolism

Glutamine synthetase deficiency

Clinical: Brain malformations, fatal neonatal multiple organ failure; static encephalopathy, recurrent hyperammonaemia; two patients so far

Diagn.:   ↓ Glutamine (serum, urine, CSF); *GS* gene

Disorders of the gamma-glutamyl cycle

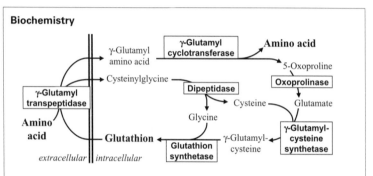

Biochemistry

The tripeptide glutathione (γ-Glu-Cys-Gly) is an essential component of cellular metabolism. It serves as a gamma-glutamyl donor for the transport of amino acids across membranes, releasing 5-oxoproline in the cytosol which is recycled to glutathione (gamma-glutamyl cycle). The sulphhydryl group of the cysteinyl residue functions as an electron donor in many reactions incl. the detoxification of oxygen radicals and organic peroxides; the resulting disulphide is regenerated in the erythrocytes by NADPH from the pentose phosphate pathway (see *page 86*). By transhydrogenation, glutathione cleaves disulphide bonds in proteins, e.g. insulin, whilst through the action of glutathione-S-transferase it binds and detoxifies various (mostly lipophilic) compounds incl. cytotoxic anticancer drugs. Glutathione is also required for the synthesis of cysteinyl leukotrienes (see also *page 165*).

Disturbances of the gamma-glutamyl cycle cause a range of clinical problems incl. *neonatal metabolic acidosis, haemolytic anaemia, electrolyte imbalances and progressive neurological symptoms.* All known enzyme defects are inherited in an aut. rec. fashion; the most important disorder in this group is glutathione synthetase deficiency. Initial investigations include the analysis of organic acids (5-oxoproline) and glutathione status in urine, erythrocytes (see *page 35*), leukocytes and/or fibroblasts. Enzyme studies are performed in erythrocytes or other nucleated cells (leukocytes, fibroblasts), but erythrocytes only contain part of the gamma-glutamyl cycle (no gamma-glutamyl transpeptidase and 5-oxoprolinase).

Gamma-glutamyl transpeptidase deficiency
Clinical: Variable; intellectual disability, psychosis; no haematological abnormalities
Diagn.:   ↑ Glutathione (urine); normal glutathione in erythrocytes, impaired synthesis of LTD_4,
            ↓ Gamma-glutamyl transpeptidase (leukocytes, fibroblasts)
Therapy: No specific treatment available

Membrane-bound dipeptidase (cysteinylglycinase) deficiency
Clinical: Intellectual disability, motor impairment, peripheral neuropathy, partial deafness
Diagn.:   ↑ Cystinylglycine (urine, plasma); glutathione status normal
Therapy: No specific treatment available

5-Oxoprolinase deficiency
Clinical: Very variable, possibly asymptomatic; single cases with intellectual disability, urolith-
            iasis, renal colic, colitis, diarrhoea
Diagn.:   OA (urine): ↑ 5-oxoproline, glutathione status normal, ↓ 5-oxoprolinase (leukocytes,
            fibroblasts); *OPLAH* gene
DD: Glutathione synthetase deficiency, secondary 5-oxoprolinuria (see above)
Therapy: None known

Gamma-glutamylcysteine synthetase deficiency
Clinical: Haemolytic anaemia, jaundice; variable: psychosis, neuropathy, ataxia, myopathy/
            muscle weakness
Diagn.:   Hyperaminoaciduria; ↓ glutathione (erythrocytes); no 5-oxoprolinuria; ↓ Gamma-
            glutamylcysteine synthetase (erythrocytes, leukocytes, fibroblasts); *GCLC* gene
Therapy: Avoid drugs that may cause haemolysis; vit. C + E may be tried

Glutathione synthetase deficiency
Clinical: *Severe form*: haemolytic anaemia, metabolic acidosis, often progressive neurological
            symptoms (e.g. intellectual disability, seizures, ataxia, spasticity)
            Mild form (erythrocytes): haemolytic anaemia
Diagn.:   OA (urine): ↑↑ 5-oxoproline; ↓ glutathione (erythrocytes, leukocytes, fibroblasts); re-
            duced synthesis of cysteinyl leukotrienes (monocytes, neutrophils, urine); ↓ glutathi-
            one synthetase (erythrocytes, fibroblasts), *GSS* gene
DD: 5-Oxoprolinase deficiency (see above); *secondary 5-oxoprolinuria:* e.g. acute decom-
            pensation in propionic aciduria, urea cycle defects, mitochondrial disorders, extreme
            prematurity, Stevens-Johnson syndrome, intoxication (e.g. paracetamol)
Therapy: Correct acidosis (Na-bicarbonate/Na-citrate/THAM), try α-tocopherol 10 mg/kg/day
            (assists granulocyte function), ascorbate (100 mg/kg/day), N-acetylcysteine, vit. E (10
            mg/kg/day); avoid drugs that may cause haemolysis (similar to glucose-6-phosphate
            dehydrogenase deficiency)

Disorders of peptide metabolism

Prolidase deficiency
Clinical: Skin lesions (ulcerations), mild intellectual disability, frequent infections
Enzyme: Prolidase = peptidase B
Bioch.: Disorder of collagen breakdown (degradation of dipeptides with N-terminal Pro/OH-Pro)
Diagn.: Peptide analysis (urine): ↑ iminodipeptides; enzyme studies; *PEPD* gene
Therapy: Symptomatic

Carnosinaemia
Clinical: May be an incidental finding
Enzyme: Carnosinase – cleaves carnosine (dipeptide β-Ala–His)
Diagn.: AA (plasma, urine): ↑ carnosine; enzyme studies
Therapy: None/none necessary

Homocarnosinosis
Clinical: Skin lesions (ulcerations), mild intellectual disability, frequent infections
Bioch.: ? Disorder of collagen breakdown
Diagn.: AA (urine); enzyme studies
Therapy: None

Carbohydrate metabolism

Biochemistry: Carbohydrate metabolism

Glucose is the most important rapid source of energy. It is catabolised to pyruvate by cytosolic glycolysis, transported into the mitochondrion and completely oxidised in the Krebs cycle, generating chemical energy. The reversible reduction of pyruvate to lactate allows anaerobic glycolysis (regenerates NAD^+). In gluconeogenesis, pyruvate is carboxylated (by *pyruvate carboxylase*, PC) to oxaloacetate which is transported via the malate shuttle into the cytosol and used for the synthesis of glucose-6-phosphate (Glc-6-P). Enzymes involved include *phosphoenolpyruvate carboxykinase* (PEPCK) and *fructose-1,6-bisphosphatase* (aldolase A). The conversion of Glc-6-P into glucose takes place in the endoplasmic reticulum and involves several transport systems in addition to the enzyme *glucose-6-phosphatase* (Glc-6-P'ase).

Glycogen, the storage form of glucose (synthesised from Glc-6-P), is especially abundant in liver (required for maintenance of normoglycaemia) and muscle (required for energy provision during exercise).

Lactose (Gal-Glc disaccharide) in milk and milk products is cleaved in the gut and absorbed. Complete oxidation of **galactose** first requires activation and conversion into UDP-glucose by galaktokinase, galactose-1-phosphate uridyltransferase (GALT) and UDP-galactose-4-epimerase, leaving the carbon structure intact. The last step is reversible and UDP-galactose can be synthesised by all cells for the glycosylation of macromolecules or to produce lactose.

Defects of galactose metabolism may cause increased production of galactitol and cataract due to its accumulation in the lens.

Fructose is a component of table sugar (sucrose, Glc-Fru disaccharide) and is contained in large amounts in fruits and various vegetables; fructose, sucrose and sorbitol (metabolised mainly via fructose) are also frequent food additives. The irreversible phosphorylation of fructose by fructokinase yields fructose-1-phosphate which is cleaved by aldolase B into phosphorylated C_3-metabolites that enter glycolysis or gluconeogenesis.

Glycerol-3-phosphate is a substrate for the synthesis of triglycerides, phospholipids, sphingolipids and other glycerolipids. It is closely linked to the glycolysis pathway via dihydroxyacetone phosphate; the glycerol-3-P dehydrogenase reaction is catalysed by different enzymes in the mitochondrion (FAD-dependent, irreversible), cytosol and peroxisome (NAD^+-dependent, reversible) and plays an important role in the transport of reducing equivalents between different cellular compartments (glycerol-3-P shuttle). Glycerol-3-P is also generated by glycerokinase-mediated activation of glycerol (resulting from glycerolipid breakdown) in liver, kidney and gut mucosa.

Disorders of galactose and fructose metabolism

Patients with a disorder of galactose or fructose metabolism develop clinical symptoms only after intake of lactose (milk, milk products) or fructose/sucrose, respectively, in the diet. The presence of reducing substances in the urine (see *page 31*) is an important first clue to the diagnosis; galactosaemia is also detected through newborn screening in many countries. Galactose-1-phosphate (Gal-1-P) and fructose-1-phosphate (Fru-1-P) which accumulate in classical galactosaemia and hereditary fructose intolerance are toxic particularly for the liver and kidneys.

Essential fructosuria

Clinical: Incidental finding, asymptomatic
Enzyme: Fructokinase (Ketohexokinase, *KHK* gene)
Therapy: None indicated

Hereditary fructose intolerance

Clinical: After weaning or supplementary fructose-containing food: vomiting, apathy, coma; progressive liver dysfunction, hepatosplenomegaly, hypoglycaemia; renal tubular dysfunction, failure to thrive, aversion to fructose-containing foods/sweets, no caries
Enzyme: Aldolase B
Genetics: *ALDOB* gene, 3 common mutations in Europeans (p.A150P [>50%], p.A175D, p.N335K; exons 5 + 9). Incidence in Europe 1:20,000
Bioch.: Toxic effect due to reduced intracellular ATP, inhibiton of glycogenolysis
Diagn.: Renal tubular damage: ↑ Glc, albumin, AA, reducing substances (urine); positive effect of withdrawing fructose; enzyme studies: liver (if mutation studies inconclusive); fructose challenge not recommended any more
Therapy: Strict fructose-restricted diet, vitamin supplements

Classical galactosaemia

Clinical: Progressive symptoms after start of milk feeds, usually starting on the 3rd or 4th day: vomiting, diarrhoea, jaundice, disturbances of liver function (most sensitive: ↓ INR), development of bilateral cataracts, sepsis (Gram-negative organisms, e.g. E. coli) → death from hepatic and renal failure

Enzyme: Galactose-1-phosphate uridyltransferase (GALT)

Genetics: *GALT* gene, common mutations p.Q188R, p.K285N; incidence in Europeans: 1:23,000–44,000.

Var.:   *Duarte 1 (D1) allele* (variants p.N314D + p.L218L) = ↑ enzyme activity
           Duarte 2 (D2) allele (p.N314D + 5'UTR deletion) = 50% enzyme activity
           Allele frequencies: D1 ~3%, D2 ~5%
           Duarte galactosaemia = compound heterozygous for null mutation + D2 variant, 25% GALT activity (variable)

Diagn.:   See *page 50* (newborn screening); GALT activity, ↑ Gal and Gal-1-P (dried blood spots, plasma, erythrocytes); galactitol (plasma, erythrocytes); renal tubular damage: ↑ Glc, albumin, AA, reducing substances (urine)

Therapy: *After* obtaining blood sample (see also *page 35*): lactose-free infant formula (may be life-saving); lactose-free, galactose-restricted diet throughout life:
           Target: Gal-1-P (erythrocytes) 2–4 mg/dl (up to 5 mg/dl – low values may be difficult to reach in early childhood due to high endogenous Gal production)
           Duarte galactosaemia: often detected on newborn screening; no evidence that it is harmful or that affected children benefit from treatment; to assure correctness of diagnosis: GALT activity in erythrocytes, mutation studies

Compl.s: Despite compliance with therapy: oro-motor/generalised dyspraxias, intellectual disability, ataxia, tremor; ovarian dysfunction with abnormal pubertal development (girls), osteoporosis

Galactokinase deficiency

Clinical: Rapidly progressive central cataract, reversible in the first weeks of life

Diagn.:   ↑ Gal, galactitol, glucose (urine), low Gal-1-P (blood); enzyme studies; *GALK1* gene

Therapy: Lactose-free diet

UDP-galactose epimerase deficiency

Clinical: *Severe (generalised)*: same as in classical galactosaemia: liver disease, failure to thrive, intellectual disability, cataracts; *benign (peripheral)*: deficiency restricted to blood cells, asymptomatic; found in newborn screening by Gal quantitation (see *page 50*)

Diagn.:   ↑ Gal and Gal-1-P (serum, erythrocytes) but normal GALT activity; enzyme studies: erythrocytes; *GALE* gene.

Therapy: Same as in classical galactosaemia (severe form)

Disorders of gluconeogenesis

A typical feature of disorders of gluconeogenesis is recurrent hypoglycaemia with lactic acidosis ± ketosis. Severe *hypoglycaemia and hepatomegaly* are found especially in enzyme defects which are close to glucose in the gluconeogenesis pathway (G6Pase [glycogen storage diseases type I; see *page 83*] and FBPase deficiencies), whilst progressive *neurodegeneration and lactic acidosis* are leading features of enzyme defects closer to the Krebs cycle (PEPCK and PC deficiencies [see pyruvate metabolism; *page 96*]).

Fructose-1,6-bisphosphatase deficiency

Clinical: Acute crisis (often neonatal) with hepatomegaly (but normal transaminases), acidosis, hyperventilation, ketosis, hypoglycaemia, coma, seizures, brain damage. Large amounts of fructose (after fasting) may lead to acute crisis.

Diagn.:   ↑ Lactate, pyruvate, ketones; OA (urine): 2-oxoglutaric acid; *FBP1* gene

Therapy: Usually responds rapidly to treatment with intravenous/oral glucose ± sodium bicarbonate

Other disorders of gluconeogenesis

• *Phosphoenolpyruvate carboxykinase deficiency*: hypotonia, hepatomegaly, failure to thrive, lactic acidosis, hypoglycaemia; unconfirmed disease entity, no molecular data.

Glycogen storage diseases (GSD, glycogenoses)

This group includes disorders of glycogen degradation (tissue-specific phosphorylases, debranching enzyme, α-glucosidase), glycolysis, glucose release, and glycogen synthesis (glycogen synthase, branching enzyme). There are three main clinical presentations:
• *Liver*: hypoglycaemia, hepatomegaly, growth retardation (GSD I, IV, VI, IX, 0)
• *Muscle*: exercise intolerance, muscle cramps (GSD V, VII; DD see *page 16*)
• *Mixed/generalised*: cardiomyopathy, liver/muscle involvement (GSD II, III)
Some conditions show mixed clinical symptoms. All GSDs except one form of type VI are aut. rec.; cumulative incidence is approx. 1:20,000. Diagnosis is confirmed by mutation analysis or biopsy (histology) and enzyme studies.

Glycogen storage disease type I (von Gierke)

Enzyme: *Type Ia*: glucose-6-phosphatase; *G6PC* gene
              Type Ib (includes former Ic and Id): glucose-6-phosphate transporter (endoplasmic reticulum); *SLC37A4* gene

Clinical: First manifestation usually at age 3–6 mths: hypoglycaemia 3–4 hrs after meals (recurrent; seizure), truncal obesity, hepatomegaly, "doll face", tachypnoea (acidosis), nephromegaly, failure to thrive, small stature

Var.:   *GSD1b*: same as above, plus neutropenia, leukocyte dysfunction, bacterial infections, diarrhoea, inflammatory bowel disease (IBD)

Diagn.:   ↓ Glucose, acidosis, ↑ lactate, severe lipaemia, ↑ triglycerides, ↑ uric acid; glucose challenge: fall in lactate; enzyme studies: liver

Therapy: Avoid hypoglycaemia by means of continuous carbohydrate intake:
              • Glucose requirement (see *page 56*)
              • Frequent meals (every 2–3 hrs in infants, 4–6 hrs in school age): slowly resorbed carbohydrates (glucose polymer/maltodextrin, starch), no sucrose, limited fructose and lactose/galactose (vegetables, fruits); soy-based milk replacement products + calcium
              • Nights: continuous (infants 12 hrs, adults 8–10 hrs) intake of glucose polymer/maltodextrin via nasogastric tube, start as soon as possible after last daytime meal; uncooked corn-starch
              Type Ib: if neutropenia/infections, add Filgrastim (G-CSF, Neupogen®), starting dose 2.5 μg/kg/day s.c. (exclude myelodysplasia by bone marrow biopsy), higher if necessary. Do not use glucocorticoids to treat IBD.

Monitor: Preprandial blood glucose > 3.5–4.0 mmol/l; urine lactate/creatinine ratio < 0.06 mmol/
            mmol; normal uric acid and liver function tests; venous blood base excess > –5 mmol/l,
            bicarbonate > 20 mmol/l; serum triglyceride concentration < 6.0 mmol/l; normal fae-
            cal α_1-antitrypsin for GSD Ib; body mass index between 0.0 and + 2.0 SDS. yearly
            ultrasound scan of the liver, check kidney function regularly (see Rake et al., Eur J
            Pediatr 2002)
Compl.s: (2nd–3rd decade): liver adenomas, anaemia, osteoporosis, renal failure

Glycogen storage disease type II (Pompe)

Enzyme: α-Glucosidase (acid maltase, *GAA* gene) → lysosomal disorder with storage of cho-
            lesterol esters and triglycerides
Clinical: *Infantile*: severe (cardio)myopathy, hypotonia, respiratory failure, failure to thrive, un-
            treated fatal in the first year
            Juvenile/adult: slowly progressive muscle weakness (only skeletal muscle); sometimes
            atherosclerosis
Diagn.:   Pathological pattern of oligosacharides (urine, probably low sensitivity); vacuolated
            lymphocytes; typical ECG (P waves, massive QRS wave and shortened PR interval)
            + echo; enzyme studies: leukocytes, dried blood spots, etc. (*caution*: neutral maltase
            may cause false negative results)
DD: Danon disease (*page 142*)
Therapy: Physiotherapy; protein-enriched nutrition with supplementation of Ala + Leu; enzyme
            replacement (alglucosidase alfa [Myozyme®, Lumizyme®])

Glycogen storage disease type III (Cori/Forbes)

Enzyme: Debranching enzyme = amylo-1,6-glucosidase, *AGL* gene (different isoforms by var-
            iant splicing: hepatic without exon 2, muscle/heart without exon 1)
Clinical: *Type IIIa* (liver + muscle): in infancy, same as in GSD type I, but normal lactate/uric
            acid; hypoglycaemias milder, improvement in childhood; normal kidney size/func-
            tion; progressive (adult) myopathy, cardiomyopathy, neuropathy
            Type IIIb: only liver manifestation
Diagn.:   ↓ Glucose; AA (plasma): ↓ Ala, Leu, Ile, Val; ↑ transaminases; ↑ cholesterol; glucose
            challenge: rise in lactate; enzyme studies: erythrocytes, fibroblasts, liver/muscle
Therapy: Maintain normoglycaemia; symptomatic treatment for myopathy; try supplementa-
            tion of alanine

Glycogen storage disease type IV (Andersen)

Enzyme: Branching enzyme = amylo-1,4 →1,6-transglucosylase; *GBE1* gene
Clinical: *Classic form*: failure to thrive, hepatomegaly, progressive liver disease → cirrhosis,
            liver failure, often fatal by age 4–5 yrs
            Mild form: non-progressive
            Neuromuscular forms: (cardio)myopathy, variable onset (prenatal-adult, incl. adult
            polyglucosan body disease [neurogenic bladder, gait difficulties, etc.])
Diagn.:   Liver/muscle biopsy: histology, electron microscopy; enzyme studies in liver/muscle
            (leukocytes, fibroblasts)
Therapy: Experimental liver transplantation

Glycogen storage disease type VI (Hers) and IX

Enzyme: *GSD type VI*: liver phosphorylase; *PYGL* gene
           GSD type IXa, b, c: phosphorylase kinase; *PHKA2* (X-linked, liver-specific), *PHKB, PHKG2* (liver-specific)
Clinical: Childhood presentation with hepatomegaly, mild hypoglycaemia, often asymptomatic; symptoms may improve with puberty, good prognosis in IXa; more severe hypoglycaemia and development of liver fibrosis/cirrhosis possible in XIb, c
Diagn.:   ↓ Glucose, ↑ lactate, ↑ transaminases; glucose challenge: rise in lactate; enzyme studies: erythrocytes (leukocytes, liver/muscle)
Therapy: Maintain normoglycaemia (uncooked cornstarch)

Glycogen storage disease type 0

No storage of glycogen
Enzyme: Glycogen synthase 2; *GYS2* gene
Clinical: Fasting: recurrent hypoglycaemia with ketosis, ↑ lactate; no organomegaly
Diagn.:   Glucose challenge: rise in lactate; glucagon challenge; enzyme studies: liver; molecular genetics
DD: Ketotic hypoglycaemia

Muscle glycogenoses

Enzymes: *GSD type V (McArdle disease)*: muscle phosphorylase; *PYGM* gene
           GSD type VII (Tarui disease): muscle phosphofructokinase; *PFKM* gene
           Muscle phosphorylase kinase: muscle-specific α-subunit; *PHKA1* (X-linked)
           Phosphoglycerate mutase 2: *PGAM2* gene
           Phosphoglucomutase 1 deficiency: *PGM1* gene
Clinical: Adolescent/adult (childhood) onset: exercise intolerance, fatigue, muscle cramps
Diagn.:   ↑ CK and uric acid (serum), myoglobinuria; muscle biopsy
Therapy: Avoid excessive exercise, creatine supplementation

Related disorders
• *Aldolase A deficiency*: childhood onset weakness, haemolytic anaemia; *ALDOA* gene
• *Enolase 3 deficiency*: single patient, adult progressive; *ENO3* gene
• *Muscle lactate dehydrogenase deficiency*: mild symptoms; *LDHM* gene
• *Muscle glycogen synthase deficiency*: childhood onset weakness, cardiomyopathy; *GYS1* gene
• *Glycogenin deficiency*: adult onset weakness, cardiac arrhythmias; *GYG1* gene
• *AMP-activated protein kinase (AMPK) deficiency*: hypertrophic cardiomyopathy (neonatal-adult onset), Wolff-Parkinson-White syndrome; *PRKAG2* gene
• *Phosphoglycerate kinase deficiency*: haemolytic anaemia, myopathy; *PGK1* gene

Fanconi-Bickel disease (glycogen storage disease type XI)

Enzyme: Glucose transporter 2; GLUT2, *SLC2A2* gene (see also *page 87*)
Clinical: Renal Fanconi syndrome, (→ rickets), aminoaciduria, phosphaturia, glucosuria, small stature, malabsorption, hepatomegaly/nephromegaly, fasting hypoglycaemia with no response to glucagon, glucose/galactose intolerance
Therapy: Frequent feeds and the use of slowly absorbed carbohydrates

Disorders of glycerol metabolism

Glycerol intolerance
Clinical: Triggered by catabolism, stress, glycerol intake: sweating, lethargy → coma, hypo-
           thermia, hypoglycaemia, sometimes seizures
Pathogen.: Unknown
Therapy: Fat-restricted (= glycerol-restricted) diet

Glycerokinase deficiency
Clinical: Recurrent vomiting, acidosis, osmotic dehydration, hypothermia, hypoglycaemia; may
           be asymptomatic (no genotype-phenotype correlation)
Genetics: *GK* gene, X-chromosomal (Xp21)
Variants: *Contiguous gene syndrome* (large deletion within Xp21 region) → congenital adrenal
           hypoplasia ± Duchenne muscular dystrophy; intellectual disability, typical facies,
           Addison disease, sometimes OTC deficiency
Diagn.:   OA (urine): ↑ glycerol (DD contamination with baby cream, etc.; may be incidental
           finding without clinical relevance); pseudohypertriglyceridaemia (if triglycerides are
           quantified by glycerol measurement after lipolysis)
Therapy: Fat-restricted (= glycerol-restricted) diet; treatment of associated conditions

Disorders of pentose/polyol metabolism

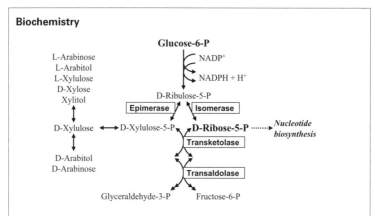

Biochemistry

The pentose phosphate pathway is required for the biosynthesis of ribose (and consequently
nucleotides) and the regeneration of NADPH/H+ from NADP+ (required for various biosyn-
thetic reactions as well as reduction of glutathione; see *page 77*). L-arabinose and xylose are
exogenous in origin (high concentration in fruit).

Disorders of the pentose phosphate pathway

These disorders can be identified by polyol analysis (urine, CSF) (NMR spectroscopy).

- *Transaldolase deficiency:* early onset liver disease, cirrhosis, hepatosplenomegaly, often fatal in infancy; haemolytic anaemia, thrombocytopenia, cardiomyopathy, renal failure; dysmorphism; fetal hydrops; diagn.: polyol analysis: ↑ ribitol, D-arabitol, erythritol, sedoheptulose; enzyme studies; *TALDO1* gene.
- *Ribose-5-P isomerase deficiency:* one patient with progressive leukoencephalopathy, ataxia, mild peripheral polyneuropathy; diagn.: MRS (brain), polyol analysis: ↑ ribitol, D-arabitol; *RPIA* gene

Pentosurias

These conditions may be accidentally discovered through a positive test of reducing substances in the urine. The exact pentose may be determined through urinary thin-layer chromatography of monosaccharides and disaccharides or gas chromatographic analysis of pentoses and polyols. Essential and alimentary pentosuria are known to be benign conditions whilst L-arabinosuria has only been described in a single patient.

- *Essential pentosuria* (L-xylulose reductase deficiency; *DCXR* gene): ↑ L-xylulose
- *Alimentary pentosuria*: ↑ xylose, arabinose (urine, plasma, CSF) after fruit ingestion
- *L-Arabinosuria* (? arabitol dehydrogenase deficiency): ↑ L-arabinose, L-arabitol

Disorders of glucose transport

A considerable number of specific transporters are involved in the transport of glucose and other monosaccharides across cellular membranes. Transporters of the GLUT family enhance passive diffusion in various tissues whilst SGLT transporters mediate active transfer coupled to an electrochemical gradient for sodium in organs where complete resorption is necessary (kidneys and intestines). GLUT transporters may be involved in the development of diabetes mellitus but conclusive evidence for this is still lacking.

GLUT1 deficiency

Glucose transport protein deficiency (epileptic encephalopathy, progressive microcephaly, mental retardatation) see page 155.

GLUT2 deficiency

Fanconi-Bickel disease (glycogen storage disease type XI) see page 85.

SGLT1 deficiency: Glucose-galactose malabsorption

Clinical: Severe neonatal diarrhoea → fluid and electrolyte imbalance, dehydration
Diagn.:   Mild glucosuria, pathological glucose/galactose tolerance tests, normal fructose tolerance test; *SLC5A1* gene
Therapy: Total parenteral nutrition; dietary replacement of glucose/galactose with fructose

SGLT2 deficiency: Renal glucosuria

Clinical: Benign glucosuria with normal blood glucose and absence of generalised or proximal tubular dysfunction; *SLC5A2* gene
Therapy: None

Congenital hyperinsulinism (CHI)

Biochemistry: Regulation of insulin secretion

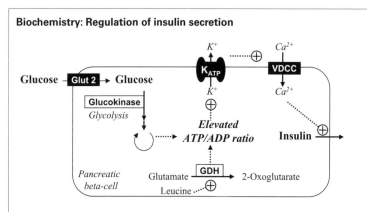

Glucose is transported by Glut2 (see also *page 85*) into the pancreatic β-cell and enters glycolysis via glucokinase (rate-limiting enzyme). The resulting increase in the ATP/ADP ratio triggers exocytosis of insulin through a complex mechanism involving closure of the K_{ATP} channel (which consists of the sulphonylurea receptor SUR1 and subunit Kir6.2), depolarisation of the cell membrane, activation of voltage-dependent calcium channels (VDCC) and calcium influx. The intracellular ATP/ADP ratio may also rise with increased oxidation of glutamate to 2-oxoglutarate mediated by glutamate dehydrogenase (GLDH). By this mechanism, leucine as an allosteric activator of GLDH may also increase insulin secretion.

Congenital hyperinsulinism (old term "nesidioblastosis") is the most common cause of persistent hypoglycaemia in early childhood (DD see *page 5*).

Congenital hyperinsulinism due to K_{ATP} channel mutations

Clinical: Neonatal hypoglycaemia, seizure, lethargy, cyanosis, large for gestational age

Genetics: Kir6.2: *KCNJ11* gene, SUR1: *ABCC8* gene, chrom. 11p15.1, imprinted region
             Diffuse form: aut. rec. or aut. dom. mutations
             Focal form: heterozygous paternal mutation, clonal loss of maternal 11p15.1

Diagn.:   ↑ Glucose requirement (up to 30 mg/kg/min)
             During hypoglycaemia (glucose <2.0 mmol/l or 40 mg/dl): ↓ ketone bodies, ↓ FFA (serum), insulin incompletely suppressed (usually >3 mU/l, not always reliable), normal blood gases and lactate, ketones (test strip) negative, n–↑ NH_3; IGFBP-1 (<120 mg/ml); normal glucagon response (rise of blood glucose >25 mg/dl)
             Important for surgical therapy: distinguish diffuse vs. focal/adenomatous forms (^{18}F-dopa positron-emission tomography; clinically indistinguishable)

DD: See below; *transient hyperinsulinism* in the neonate (diabetic fetopathy, asphyxia, sepsis, rhesus incompatibility, SGA, etc.); hypopituitarism

Therapy: Central line, high *glucose* infusion (10–25 mg/kg/min). Aggressive treatment to avoid repeated hypoglycaemia is essential for good developmental outcome!

- *Diazoxide* (10–15 mg/kg/day in 3 doses); effect usually within up to 5 days, may cause severe cardiac failure, fluid retention, leukopenia; consider additional hydrochlorothiazide (1–2 mg/kg/day in 2 doses)
  Caution: high number (95%) of diazoxide non-responders, especially in neonates
- Alternative: *octreotide* (5–20 µg/kg/day s.c. in 3–4 doses) may cause tachyphylaxis
- Acute situations: *glucagon* (1–4 mg/day [5–10 µg/kg/hr] i.v.) continuously over 2–3 days
- Trial with *nifedipine* (0.5–2 mg/kg/day) may be justified in selected cases.

If conservative therapy is ineffective: subtotal-total pancreatic resection (90–95%); *focal form*: selective resection of insulin-producing adenoma

Other disorders associated with congenital hyperinsulinism

- *Glucokinase activating mutations* (*GCK* gene, aut. dom.): good response to diazoxide (GCK loss of function mutations cause [heterozygous] familial mild non-progressive hyperglycaemia, gestational diabetes, [homozygous] neonatal diabetes)
- *Hyperinsulinism-hyperammonaemia syndrome* (glutamate dehydrogenase activating mutations, *GLDH* gene, aut. dom.): hyperammonaemia 100–200 µmol/l, usually asymptomatic, may be prominent early but may disappear later in childhood; often leucine-sensitive; therapy: consider protein-restricted diet, good response to diazoxide
- *Exercise-induced hyperinsulinaemic hypoglycaemia*: children/adults with syncopal episodes after exercise. *SLC16A1* promoter mutations (monocarboxylate transporter 1, aut. dom.) causing abnormal pyruvate uptake into pancreatic β-cells.
- *Short-chain hydroxyacyl-CoA dehydrogenase (SCHAD) deficiency* (*HADH* gene, aut. rec.): intermittent unpredictable hypoglycaemia with seizures, good effect of diazoxide; acylcarnitines: ↑ $C_{4\text{-OH}}$-carnitine; OA (urine): ↑ 3-OH-glutarate
- *Phosphomannose isomerase deficiency*: CDG type Ib (see *page 148*)
- *Beckwith-Wiedemann syndrome*: typical face, macroglossia, ear creases, omphalocele, visceromegaly, hemihypertrophy; diffuse hyperinsulinism, disappears in most patients within weeks; chromosomal imbalance 11p15 (e.g. paternal UPD)

Fatty acid and ketone body metabolism

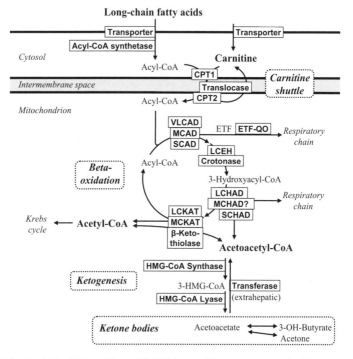

Biochemistry: Fatty acid oxidation and the metabolism of ketone bodies

Mitochondrial oxidation of fatty acids (FA) is one of the major sources of cellular energy, providing up to 80% of the total requirement during fasting. The brain is unable to fully oxidise fatty acids but can adapt to the catabolism of ketone bodies synthesised by the liver. During fasting or prolonged exercise, long-chain fatty acids (C_{16}–C_{20}) stored as triglycerides in fat tissue are released by lipases and activated to acyl-CoA esters. The inner mitochondrial membrane is not permeable to long-chain fatty acids which are transported into the mitochondria via the carnitine shuttle. Carnitine is transported into cells (incl. renal tubular epithelial cells) by a high affinity carnitine transporter. Several chain-length specific enzymes shorten acyl-CoA by two carbon atoms (one acetyl-CoA) in subsequent β-oxidation cycles. Most of the long-chain specific enzymes are associated with the inner mitochondrial membrane, while medium and short-chain enzymes localise to the mitochondrial matrix. Acetyl-CoA enters the tricarboxylic acid (TCA) cycle or is converted to ketone bodies. Protons generated by dehydrogenases are transferred to the respiratory chain. Extrahepatic ketolysis requires succinyl-CoA:3-oxoacid CoA-transferase (SCOT).

Enzyme abbreviations: see description of individual disorders

Disorders of fatty acid oxidation and ketogenesis

Clinical features

Disorders of fatty acid oxidation and ketogenesis can present with great variability. Insufficient ketone body production in combination with inhibition of gluconeogenesis by low acetyl-CoA during catabolic states (prolonged fasting, surgery, infection, etc.) may cause the typical *hypoketotic hypoglycaemic coma* which may be accompanied by signs of *liver failure* with hyperammonaemia. The first manifestation is freqently in late infancy. Accumulation of toxic long-chain acylcarnitines particularly in long-chain fatty acid oxidation disorders may cause *severe neonatal lactic acidosis, cardiomyopathy and hepatopathy* resembling a respiratory chain defect. Milder deficiency variants of long-chain fatty acid oxidation and the carnitine shuttle may affect *skeletal muscle* and become manifest in adolescence or early adulthood as chronic weakness, pain or recurrent rhabdomyolysis, or cause acute or chronic *cardiomyopathies*. The renal excretion of large amounts of acylcarnitines can lead to secondary carnitine deficiency. In many countries, fatty acid oxidation defects are identified through tandem mass spectrometry in newborn screening programmes. Not surprisingly, when identified presymptomatically, many of the disorders have a mild phenotype. However, patients with the long chain enzyme defects often still have chronic symptoms, albeit milder, in spite of diagnosis through newborn screening. All disorders in this group are inherited in an aut. rec. fashion though heterozygotes can occasionally express symptoms.

Diagnosis

The simultaneous determination of serum concentrations of free fatty acids and ketones (3-hydroxybutyrate) is essential for rapid recognition of fatty acid oxidation disorders in acute hypoglycaemia. Acylcarnitine analysis is usually diagnostic; normal results despite hypoketotic hypoglycaemia may be suggestive of HMG-CoA synthase deficiency. Organic acid analyses and serum carnitine studies may be helpful. Enzyme studies (leukocytes, fibroblasts) and molecular studies confirm the diagnoses and allow linkage investigations. Challenge tests (fasting test, oil challenge) are indicated only in selected, exceptional cases and should only be carried out in specialised metabolic centres (danger of acute cardiotoxicity and other complications!).

- *Acute*: see *page 5* – investigations during symptomatic hypoglycaemia
- *Clinical chemistry*: ↓ Glc, n–↑ liver enzymes, NH₃, lactate, CK, myoglobin
- *Free fatty acids and ketones* (plasma, serum): normal values see *page 167*
- *Carnitine status* (serum): ↓ total carnitine (may be elevated in acute crisis), ↑ acylcarnitine/total carnitine ratio; in CPT1 deficiency ↑ free and total carnitine, ↓ acylcarnitine
- *Acylcarnitines* (filter paper card, plasma): specific metabolites, rapid diagnosis, but carnitine transporter deficiency may give borderline results
- *Organic acids* (urine): specific dicarboxylic acids arising from microsomal ω-oxidation of fatty acids; specific acylglycines in some disorders; ketones (test strip) not always negative
- *Enzyme studies* (fibroblasts, lymphocytes)
- *Molecular studies* may be helpful in several disorders, particularly MCAD and LCHAD deficiencies (common mutations) (common SCAD variants may explain elevated urinary ethylmalonic acid; see *page 64*).
- *Histology:* often fatty degeneration, lipid myopathy

Treatment

- *Avoid fasting*, early intervention in gastroenteritis, etc.
- **Acute**: high dose *glucose* i.v. (7–10 mg/kg/min), if necessary add insulin, keep blood glucose at 5.5 mmol/l (100 mg/dl). Excessive glucose may increase lactic acidosis.
- Do not give intravenous lipids.
- **In proven disorders of long-chain fatty acid oxidation and the carnitine cycle:**
  acute: dialysis, exchange transfusion; medium-chain triglyceride via NG-tube or G-tube as slow continuous drip as needed
  long-term: medium-chain triglycerides; experimental: D,L-3-hydroxybutyrate
- In ETF or ETF dehydrogenase deficiencies: try riboflavin 150 mg/day
- Persisting severe reduction of serum carnitine: consider carnitine supplementation (up to 50–100 mg/kg/day); may be detrimental in disorders of long-chain fatty acid oxidation or the carnitine cycle (long-chain acylcarnitines are cardiotoxic); not usually necessary for MCAD deficiency

Carnitine transporter deficiency
(primary carnitine deficiency, carnitine uptake deficiency)

Clinical: Cardiomyopathy, arrhythmias, cardiac failure, muscle weakness, liver disease; may be asymptomatic (mothers in newborn screening)

Bioch.:   Intracellular carnitine deficiency (muscle), carnitine depletion due to deficient renal reabsorption

Diagn.:   Serum: $\downarrow\downarrow\downarrow$ free/total carnitine (<5–10% normal); urine: calculate fractional tubular re-absorption of free carnitine (normal >98%; acylcarnitines: usually $\downarrow\downarrow$ all compounds; OA (urine): no (few) dicarboxylic acids; *SLC22A5* gene

Therapy: Carnitine 100 mg/kg/day, check serum levels to monitor compliance; long-term ECG, consider implantation of defibrillator

Carnitine palmitoyltransferase I (CPT1) deficiency

Clinical: Same as above, severe liver disease, no (cardio)myopathy; renal tubular acidosis; mild variant of unknown clinical relevance in some populations

Diagn.:   Carnitine status: n–$\uparrow$ total/free carnitine, <20% acylcarnitine; acylcarnitines: n–$\uparrow$ free carnitine, $\downarrow$ C_{16}, C_{18}, $C_{18:1}$; OA (urine): no dicarboxylic aciduria; *CPT1A* gene

Carnitine translocase (carnitine acylcarnitine carrier) deficiency

Clinical: Same as above, severe cardiomyopathy, arrhythmias, liver disease; most reported cases have proven lethal in the first year of life

Diagn.:   Serum: $\downarrow\downarrow$ total carnitine, 80–100% acylcarnitine; acylcarnitines: $\uparrow\uparrow$ C_{16}, C_{18}, $C_{18:1}$, $\downarrow$ free carnitine; OA (urine): ± dicarboxylic aciduria; *SLC25A20* gene

Carnitine palmitoyltransferase II (CPT2) deficiency

Clinical: *Early onset form*: as above, cardiomyopathy, liver disease
            Attenuated form: adult onset episodic muscle weakness, exercise intolerance (DD *page 16*), rhabdomyolysis (e.g. during fever); *intermediate forms*

Diagn.:   Serum: $\downarrow$ total carnitine, 40–80% acylcarnitine; acylcarnitines: $\uparrow$ ratio $(C_{16} + C_{18:1})/(C_2)$; OA (urine): no/non-specific dicarboxylic acids; *CPT2* gene

(Very) long-chain acyl-CoA dehydrogenase (VLCAD) deficiency

Clinical: *Severe form*: as above, cardiomyopathy, liver disease, hepatomegaly, SIDS; *attenuated form*: late onset recurrent rhabdomyolysis, exercise intolerance

Diagn.:   Acylcarnitines: ↑ $C_{14:1}$, ratio $C_{14:1}/C_{12:1}$; OA (urine): C_6–C_{14} dicarboxylic acids; *ACADVL* gene

Therapy: *Attenuated form*: same as in MCAD deficiency; *severe form*: same as in LCHAD deficiency

Mitochondrial trifunctional protein (MTP) deficiency, long-chain hydroxyacyl-CoA dehydrogenase (LCHAD) deficiency

MTP consists of 4 α-subunits (*HADHA* gene) mediating hydratase (LCEH) and dehydrogenase (LCHAD) activities, and 4 β-subunits (*HADHB* gene) mediating oxothiolase (LCKAT) activity. LCHAD function is primarily affected in the majority of patients (common *HADHA* mutation p.E510Q).

Clinical: Same as above, cardiomyopathy, liver disease, muscular hypotonia, neuropathy, retinopathy; late onset recurrent rhabdomyolysis; mothers of an affected fetus may develop steatosis or HELLP syndrome in pregnancy

Diagn.:   ↑ Lactate (3-hydroxypalmitoyl-CoA inhibits PDH); acylcarnitines: ↑ Hydroxy compounds $C_{14\text{-OH}}$, $C_{16\text{-OH}}$, $C_{18\text{-OH}}$, $C_{18:1\text{-OH}}$; OA (urine): C_6–C_{14} (hydroxy)dicarboxylic acids; common mutation p.E510Q

Therapy: Dietary therapy: medium-chain triglycerides, ↓ long-chain fatty acids; frequent meals, avoid fasting for >4–6 hrs in infancy, 8 hrs in older children, carnitine supplementation may be harmful

Medium-chain acyl-CoA dehydrogenase (MCAD) deficiency

MCAD deficiency is the most common fatty acid oxidation disorder in Northern Europe (incidence up to 1:6,000) due to a prevalent mutation p.K329E in the *ACADM* gene. It is now included in most newborn screening programs.

Clinical: Reye-like, often rapidly progressive metabolic crisis after 8–12–16 hrs fasting (shorter time in infants), during ordinary illness, after surgery, etc.: lethargy, nausea, vomiting (often with normal blood sugar) → within 1–2 hrs coma, seizures, cardiac arrest; no primary muscle involvement, frequently asymtopmatic

Var.:   *Mild form* frequently found by newborn screening (associated with mutation p.Y67H), of uncertain clinical relevance

Diagn.:   Acylcarnitines: ↑ C_8, C_6, ↑ ratio C_8/C_{10}; OA (urine): C_6–C_{10} dicarboxylic acids, suberylglycine, hexanoylglycine; mutation analysis (p.K329E)

Therapy: Avoidance of fasting; normal feeding intervals are safe when the child/adult is well; consider low-dose carnitine if free carnitine is very low

Progn.:   Excellent after diagnosis; most children identified through newborn screening remain without long term sequelae. Historically, a first crisis in an undiagnosed patient has been fatal in up to 25% of cases; often residual neurological damage.

Short-chain β-oxidation disorders

- *Short-chain acyl-CoA dehydrogenase (SCAD) deficiency (ACADS* gene): possible non-disease – patients with complete deficiency recognised in newborn screening ($\uparrow$ C_4 acylcarnitines) usually remain asymptomatic; mild form caused by two common polymorphisms, may explain mild ethylmalonic aciduria (see *page 64*)
- *Short-chain hydroxyacyl-CoA dehydrogenase (SCHAD) deficiency*: see *page 89*; hyperinsulinaemic hypoglycaemia

Multiple acyl-CoA dehydrogenase deficiency (glutaric aciduria type II)

Deficient electron transfer from the FAD-dependent dehydrogenases to the respiratory chain due to genetic defects of the electron transfer flavoprotein (ETF; α- and β-subunits, *ETFA* and *ETFB* genes) or ETF-coenzyme Q-oxidoreductase (ETF-QO, *ETFDH* gene); does not only affect fatty acid oxidation but also dehydrogenases involved in the metabolism of amino acids (e.g. Val, Leu, Ile, Trp, Lys).

Clinical:	Facial and cerebral malformations, cystic renal disease, Reye syndrome, metabolic acidosis, hypoglycaemia, progressive encephalopathy, epilepsy, (cardio)myopathy; frequent milder/myopathic variants, riboflavin responsive (*ETFDH* mutations)
Diagn.:	Acylcarnitines: $\uparrow$ all compounds C_4–C_{18}; OA (urine): $\uparrow$ lactic, glutaric, ethylmalonic, dicarboxylic acids, etc.; enzyme studies; mutations mostly *ETFA*
Therapy:	Avoidance of fasting; low-fat diet; try riboflavin 150 mg/day; experimental: D-3-hydroxybutyrate
Progn.:	Neonatal presentation usually fatal in the first weeks of life

HMG-CoA synthase deficiency

Clinical:	Acute hypoketotic hypoglycaemia, relatively short fasting tolerance
Diagn.:	OA (fasting urine): dicarboxylic aciduria without ketosis; $\uparrow$ 4-hydroxy-6-methyl-2-pyrone; normal acylcarnitines; normal metabolic studies outside fasting; *HMGCS2* mutation studies; (enzyme studies no option)
Therapy:	Same as in fatty acid oxidation defects
Progn.:	Excellent when fasting is avoided

HMG-CoA lyase deficiency

3-Hydroxy-3-methylglutaryl-(HMG-)CoA lyase is required for ketogenesis but also performs the final step in the leucine degradative pathway (see *page 60*).

Clinical:	Acute hypoketotic hypoglycaemia, metabolic acidosis, liver disease, often fatal with Reye-like crisis
Diagn.:	OA (urine): specific metabolites (3-HMG, 3-methylglutaconic acid, etc.); *HMGCL* gene
Therapy:	*Acute*: same as in organic acidurias (see *page 56*), carnitine, high-dose glucose i.v. *Long-term*: low-fat (approx. 25% of daily energy requirement) protein-restricted diet, carnitine substitution
Progn.:	Good, if no residual damage from first manifestation

Disorders of ketolysis

For the differential diagnosis of ketosis see *page 11*. Failure to utilise ketone bodies synthesised in the liver causes severe ketoacidosis and *hyper*ketotic hypoglycaemia.

Succinyl-CoA:3-oxoacid-CoA transferase (SCOT) deficiency

Clinical: Recurrent episodes of severe ketoacidosis, tachypnoea, hypotonia, coma

Manif.: Neonatal period or infancy

Diagn.: ↑ Ketones (D-3-hydroxybutyrate) in serum and urine, persistent in fed state, excessive in fasting; mutation studies, enzyme studies; OA (urine): ↑ ketones, otherwise non-specific; acylcarnitines normal; *SCOT* gene

3-Oxothiolase (mitochondrial acetoacetyl-CoA lyase) deficiency

This enzyme is required for ketolysis but also performs the final step in the isoleucine degradative pathway (see *page 60*).

Clinical: Acute episodes of nausea, vomiting, → coma, residual neurological abnormalities

Diagn.: ↑ Ketones (D-3-hydroxybutyrate) in serum and urine, relatively high blood glucose, (lactic) acidosis, n–↑ NH_3; acylcarnitines: tiglylcarnitine, 2-methyl-3-hydroxybutyl-carnitine and others; OA (urine): ↑ 2-methyl-3-hydroxybutyrate, 2-methylacetoacetate, tiglylglycine; consider Ile challenge (100 mg/kg, collect urine for 8 hrs → OA); *ACAT1* gene

Energy metabolism

Disorders that affect the cellular supply of ATP disturb numerous functions especially in organs with a high energy requirement such as brain, skeletal muscle, heart, liver, kidney or retina. Patients show various *combinations of neuromuscular and other symptoms* involving *different, independent organ systems*, sometimes explained by tissue-specific expression of a particular genetic defect. The *disease course* is variable but often *rapidly progressive*. There is some overlap with cerebral organic acidurias (*page 61*). In a few cases there is only single organ involvement (e.g. muscle, heart, liver).

Mitochondrial disorders in a strict sense are disorders of enzymes or enzyme complexes directly involved in the generation of chemical energy by oxidative phosphorylation. These include disorders of pyruvate metabolism and the Krebs (tricarboxylic acid) cycle as well as the respiratory chain and ATP synthase. There is considerable overlap between individual disorders with regard to clinical features, pathophysiology and genetics as some proteins are shared by several enzyme complexes and accumulating metabolites may have an inhibitory effect on other enzymes. Blockage of the respiratory chain due to O_2 deficiency, genetic defects or inhibitors causes a rise in the $NADH/NAD^+$ ratio which in turn inhibits PDH and other enzymes of intermediary metabolism incl. the Krebs cycle.

Disorders of pyruvate metabolism and the Krebs cycle

Biochemistry: Pyruvate metabolism and the Krebs cycle

Pyruvate is mostly formed from glycolysis and can be reversibly converted by LDH to lactate (the end product of anaerobic glycolysis) or by ALAT to alanine (the corresponding amino acid). It is metabolised irreversibly either by pyruvate carboxylase (gluconeogenesis and anaplerosis of the Krebs cycle) and the pyruvate dehydrogenase complex (formation of acetyl-CoA which is metabolised in the Krebs cycle). Thus this metabolite lies at a critical junction in intermediary metabolism. The *Krebs cycle* (tricarboxylic acid cycle) converts acetyl-CoA to carbon dioxide and energy in the form of GTP and reduced cofactors (NADH and $FADH_2$).

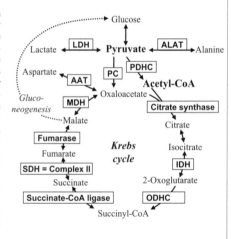

Abbreviations: AAT = aspartate aminotransferase, ALAT = alanine aminotransferase, IDH = isocitrate dehydrogenase, LDH = lactate dehydrogenase, MDH = malate dehydrogenase, ODHC = 2-oxoglutarate dehydrogenase complex, PDHC = pyruvate dehydrogenase complex, PC = pyruvate carboxylase

Pyruvate dehydrogenase (PDH) deficiency

Multi-subunit enzyme complex with the following components (genes in parentheses):

- *E1* = decarboxylase, heterotetramer of two proteins E1α (*PDHA1*) and E1β (*PDHB*)
- *E2* = dihydrolipoamide acetyltransferase (*DLAT*)
- *E3* = dihydrolipoamide dehydrogenase (*DLD*); also component of the α-ketoglutarate dehydrogenase and the branched-chain α-ketoacid dehydrogenase complexes
- *E3BP* = E3-binding protein, protein X (*PDHX*)
- *Cofactors*: thiamine pyrophosphate, α-lipoic acid, FAD, NAD$^+$ and CoA

Regulation: PDH activity is inactivated through phosphorylation by specific PDH kinases (*PDK1–4*) and reactivated (dephosphorylated) by PDH phosphatases (*PDP1–2, PDPR*).

Genetics:	Most common form is X-chromosomal (*PDHA1* gene) → boys are more frequently affected than girls
Clinical:	Global developmental delay, hypotonia, epilepsy, ataxia (may be intermittent), apnoea, progressive encephalopathy (incl. Leigh or Leigh-like syndrome, focal brain stem lesions); acute peripheral neuropathy, brain malformations; congenital lactic acidosis
Variants:	*E2 (dihydrolipoamide acetyltransferase) deficiency*: symmetric necrotic lesions in the globus pallidus, dystonia
	E3 (dihydrolipoamide dehydrogenase) deficiency: developmental delay, hypotonia; Leigh syndrome; lactic acidosis plus biochemical findings of maple syrup urine disease (elevated plasma leucine, isoleucine and valine – *page 66*)
Diagn.:	↑ Lactate, pyruvate, alanine in body fluids, n–↓ lactate/pyruvate ratio; enzyme assay in fibroblasts; immunoblot to determine which subunit is deficient
Therapy:	Ketogenic diet (3:1–5:1), thiamine (150–300 mg/day)
Progn.:	Often poor, depending on severity of the deficiency

Pyruvate carboxylase deficiency

The synthesis of oxaloacetate from pyruvate is not only necessary for gluconeogenesis from lactate or alanine, it also mediates anaplerosis of the Krebs cycle, i.e. replacement of citrate, 2-oxoglutarate or succinyl-CoA used for biosynthesis of various compounds, and is required for the synthesis of aspartate which is used in the transport of reducing equivalents across the mitochondrial membrane and in the urea cycle.

Clinical:	*Type A ("North American")*: developmental delay, lactic acidosis
	Type B ("French"): congenital lactic acidosis, hypotonia, encephalopathy, coma, seizures, mild hypoglycaemia, renal tubular acidosis; fatal in infancy
	Type C ("benign"): episodes of lactic acidosis + hypoglycaemia, normal development
Diagn.:	↑ Lactate, pyruvate, ketones, NH$_3$; n–↑ lactate/pyruvate ratio but ↓ 3-OH-butyrate/acetoacetate ratio; AA (plasma): ↑ Cit, Ala, Lys, Pro; OA (urine): 2-oxoglutaric acid, etc.; enzyme assay (fibrobl.); *PC* gene
DD:	Multiple carboxylase deficiency (see *page 159*)
Therapy:	No effective treatment known for variants A and B; supportive treatment for episodes of hypoglycaemia and acute lactic acidosis important in variant C

2-Oxoglutarate dehydrogenase complex (ODHC) deficiency
2-Oxoglutarate (also: α-ketoglutarate) is not only an integral metabolite in the Krebs cycle but is also a substrate for glutamate biosynthesis and has various cellular signalling functions. It consists of three proteins: E1k (*OGDH* gene), E2k (*DLST* gene) and E3 (see PDHC). ODHC deficiency is rare; so far only E3 mutations have been reported.

Clinical: Hypotonia, progressive encephalopathy with pyramidal signs, congenital lactic acidosis; mostly poor prognosis

Diagn.: OA (urine): ↑ α-ketoglutaric acid (NB: α-ketoglutaric aciduria also seen in some mitochondrial respiratory chain disorders); enzyme assay (fibroblasts)

Fumarase deficiency (fumaric aciduria):
Genetics: Aut. rec. fumarate hydratase (*FH*) deficiency: systemic childhood disease; *heterozygotes*: tumour disposition (clonal loss of second allele)

Clinical: *Systemic deficiency*: progressive encephalopathy, sometimes prenatal onset (polyhydramnios, brain malformations), prematurity, dysmorphism, hypotonia, seizures, micro-/macrocephaly, congenital lactic acidosis
Heterozygotes: multiple cutaneous and uterine leiomyomas (MCUL); hereditary leiomyomatosis and renal cell cancer (HLRCC)

Diagn.: OA (urine): ↑↑ fumarate (NB also seen in some mitochondrial respiratory chain disorders); enzyme studies (fibroblasts)

Other disorders of the Krebs cycle
* *Succinate-CoA ligase deficiency*: mutations in *SUCLA2* and *SUCLG1* lead to mitochondrial DNA depletion syndromes (MDDS; *page 106*) with mild methylmalonic aciduria
* *Succinate dehydrogenase (SDH) deficiency*: → respiratory chain complex II (*page 110*)
* *Combined aconitase and SDH deficiency*: (Swedish-type) myopathy and exercise intolerance; *ISCU* gene (deficient iron sulphur cluster scaffold protein)
* *Isocitrate dehydrogenase*: *IDH1*: cytosolic; *IDH2*: mitochondrial NADP$^+$-specific, heterozygous mutations cause D-2-hydroxyglutaric aciduria (see *page 64*) (somatic *IDH1* and *IDH2* mutations also found in gliomas and acute myeloid leukaemia); *IDH3*: mitochondrial NAD$^+$-specific, mutations cause aut. rec. retinitis pigmentosa

Mitochondrial respiratory chain disorders

Biochemistry: Mitochondrial respiratory chain

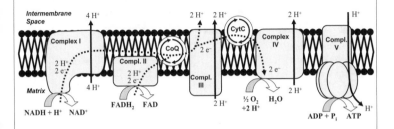

	Complex I	Complex II	Complex III	Complex IV	Complex V
mtDNA	7 Subunits		1 Subunit	3 Subunits	2 Subunits
nDNA	38 Subunits	4 Subunits	10 Subunits	10 Subunits	14 Subunits

Mitochondria are dynamic subcellular organelles with multiple functions, incl. production of ATP via the respiratory chain (RC = complexes I–IV) and oxidative phosphorylation system (OXPHOS = complexes I–V), generation of reactive oxygen species (ROS), intracellular calcium homeostasis, and critical roles in programmed cell death (apoptosis). NADH originates mostly from the Krebs cycle and is oxidised by complex I, whilst $FADH_2$ is generated e.g. through beta-oxidation of fatty acids and is oxidised by complex II. The redox reactions in complexes I, III and IV generate a proton gradient across the inner mitochondrial membrane that drives ATP synthase (= complex V). *Abbreviations*: CoQ = ubiquinone (coenzyme Q), CytC = cytochrome C, mtDNA/nDNA = mitochondrial/nuclear DNA.

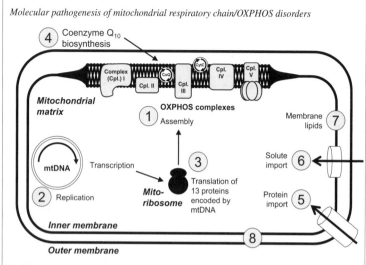

Molecular pathogenesis of mitochondrial respiratory chain/OXPHOS disorders

1. Disorders of OXPHOS complexes or their assembly
2. Disorders of mitochondrial DNA (mtDNA) maintenance
3. Disorders of mitochondrial translation
4. Disorders of coenzyme Q_{10} biosynthesis
5. Disorders of mitochondrial protein import, e.g. deafness-dystonia syndrome
6. Disorders of mitochondrial solute import, e.g. phosphate carrier deficiency
7. Disorders of mitochondrial membrane lipids, e.g. Barth syndrome
8. Disorders of the motility of mitochondrial membranes

Disorders of the mitochondrial RC/OXPHOS are clinically, biochemically and genetically hetero-geneous. The minimal birth prevalence is thought to be ~1 in 5,000, but ~1 in 250 people have a pathogenic mtDNA mutation. Classification of mitochondrial disease may be according to clini-cal features, enzyme defect(s), or the specific molecular genetic defect. Various diagnostic rating scales have been devised but diagnosis remains challenging and difficult to prove in many cases. Some characteristic clinical syndromes are recognised but many patients do not fit neatly into one of these syndromes but instead have 'overlap' symptoms/signs with features of more than one 'classical' syndrome. The range of possible symptoms/signs in mitochondrial disease is very di-verse (see table below) and it is often the involvement of two or more seemingly unrelated organs/tissues that leads to the suspicion of a mitochondrial disorder.

RC/OXPHOS disorders can present at any age. Intra-uterine development may be affected, result-ing in intrauterine growth retardation and (cerebral) malformations at birth. Young children fre-quently suffer from encephalomyopathic disease whilst myopathies predominate in the adult. Symptoms are often progressive, but can be relatively static for long periods of time. RC/OXPHOS disorders in children are often due to mutations in nuclear genes for subunits or assembly factors (described for all complexes) which usually present within the first 5 yrs of life. Mitochondrial DNA (mtDNA) mutations, often inherited in variable distribution from the mother, are more fre-quently associated with specific clinical syndromes and often present at a later age.

Clinical features

The clinical evaluation of a suspected mitochondrial disorder should entail: (a) full assessment of muscle function incl. creatine kinase and possibly muscle ultrasound (consider EMG); (b) full neurological examination; (c) detailed assessment of the function of other organ systems.

Organ/tissue	Symptoms
General/systemic	Intrauterine growth retardation, failure to thrive, small stature, lactic acidosis, hypoglycaemia
Central nervous system	Acute encephalopathy, seizures, hypotonia, hypertonia, dystonia, cerebellar ataxia, developmental delay and regression, migraine, stroke-like episodes
Ear/eye	Sensorineural hearing loss, auditory neuropathy, ptosis and progressive external ophthalmoplegia (PEO), cataract/corneal opacities, optic atrophy, pigmentary retinopathy
Neuromuscular	Muscle weakness, exercise intolerance, rhabdomyolysis, peripheral neuropathy (axonal or demyelinating)
Cardiac	Cardiomyopathy (usually hypertrophic [HCM] but can be dilated [DCM] or non-compaction), conduction defects
Endocrine	Diabetes mellitus, growth hormone insufficiency, adrenal insufficiency, hypothyroidism, hypoparathyroidism
Gastrointestinal/liver	Vomiting, chronic diarrhoea, intestinal pseudo-obstruction; exocrine pancreatic dysfunction; hepatomegaly, liver dysfunction, fulminant liver failure
Renal	Proximal tubulopathy, tubulointerstitial nephritis; steroid-resistant nephrotic syndrome with focal segmental glomerulosclerosis (primary coenzyme Q_{10} deficiency)
Haematopoietic	Sideroblastic anaemia, neutropenia, thrombocytopenia, pancytopaenia
Skin/hair	Hypertrichosis

A mitochondrial disorder should be strongly considered in patients with:
- Muscle disease and involvement of two additional systems, as described above (one of which may be CNS)
- CNS disease and involvement of two additional systems, as described above (one of which may be muscle)
- Multi-system disease (at least three systems) which may include involvement of muscle and/or CNS

Investigations

There is no single diagnostic test for mitochondrial disease, so a range of approaches are needed to try to confirm a diagnosis.

Metabolic investigations
- *Lactic acid in plasma or blood* – measure on several occasions, incl. pre- and post-prandial samples; elevated levels are a helpful diagnostic clue but normal levels do not exclude mitochondrial disease; beware artefactual elevation (screaming/struggling child or excessive squeez-

ing to obtain blood sample); lactate may also be elevated in hypoxia, after seizures and with certain drugs (e.g. ethanol, metformin)
- *Lactate:pyruvate ratio* – normal ratio e.g. in PDH deficiency; only reliable if lactate is elevated and sample is immediately deproteinised (e.g. in perchloric acid) at bedside
- *CSF lactate* – may be elevated, particularly where there is CNS involvement; normal level does not exclude mitochondrial disease
- *Plasma amino acids* – alanine may be elevated (reflecting transamination of elevated pyruvate); suggests persistent lactic acidosis; may be the only biochemical clue to mitochondrial disease in some patients with normal blood lactate levels
- *CSF amino acids* – alanine may be elevated (as in plasma)
- *CSF protein* – may be elevated, e.g. in KSS
- *CSF neurotransmitters* – 5-methyltetrahydrofolate (5MTHF) may be low, e.g. in Kearns-Sayre syndrome (KSS)
- *Acylcarnitine profile* – elevated succinylcarnitine and propionylcarnitine in *SUCLA2* and *SUCLG1* defects
- *Urine organic acids* – lactic aciduria (and related metabolites); methylmalonic aciduria with *SUCLA2* and *SUCLG1* mutations; 3-methylglutaconic aciduria in Barth syndrome and other conditions (*page 63*)
- *Biotinidase* – should be measured in all cases with lactic acidosis, since deficiency is treatable with biotin

Specialised tests
- *Peripheral blood mononuclear cell coenzyme Q_{10}* – may be useful screen for disorders of coenzyme Q_{10} biosynthesis, but may be secondarily reduced in other mitochondrial disorders
- *Plasma/urine thymidine and deoxyuridine* – elevated in MNGIE syndrome
- *Thymidine phosphorylase* (assayed in platelets or leukocytes) – deficient in MNGIE syndrome
- *Tetralinoleoyl cardiolipin* (in platelets) – Barth syndrome

Systems screen (consider investigations in parentheses)
Thorough investigation of suspected mitochondrial disease should include a search for multi-system disease, incl. specialised ophthalmological, audiological and cardiac assessment, as well as evaluation of liver, renal tubular and endocrine function.
- *Blood* (check blood count, reticulocytes): sideroblastic anaemia, pancytopenia
- *Gastrointestinal tract* (check liver enzymes, amylase, lipase, bilirubin, coagulation): acute or chronic hepatic dysfunction, failure to thrive, exocrine pancreatic dysfunction ($\downarrow$ elastase in stool; >7% fat excretion), intestinal pseudo-obstruction, otherwise unexplained chronic diarrhoea (>3 wks)
- *Endocrine* (check blood glucose and screen for deficiencies of thyroid, parathyroid, adrenal and growth hormones): short stature, delayed puberty, diabetes mellitus, central diabetes insipidus
- *Heart (*check ECG, echocardiography): cardiomyopathy (in the absence of a congenital heart defect or hypertension), conduction defect
- *Kidney* (check urea, creatinine, renal tubular function): proximal tubular dysfunction (Fanconi syndrome), focal segmental glomerulosclerosis
- *Eyes* (full ophthalmological examination, consider ERG): cataract, retinopathy, optic atrophy
- *Hearing* (assessment by audiologist): sensorineural hearing loss, auditory neuropathy
- *Peripheral nerves* (clinical examination; check neurophysiology in case of clinical suspicion): peripheral neuropathy (axonal or demyelinating)
- *General*: exacerbation of listed symptoms or signs with minor illness; sudden unexplained neonatal or infantile death in family history, feeding difficulties, generally "not well"

Neuroradiological studies
- *MRI* may reveal bilateral symmetrical T2-weighted hyperintense lesions in putamina, globi pallidi, caudate nuclei and brain stem in Leigh or Leigh-like syndrome; or stroke-like lesions (often parieto-occipital, not confined to a vascular territory) in MELAS syndrome. Appearances may fluctuate over time. MRI appearances in patients with mitochondrial disease are often non-specific and include leukodystrophy and cerebral or cerebellar atrophy. Characteristic lesions may be recognised in three genetic defects:
  - Leukoencephalopathy with brain stem and spinal cord involvement and lactate accumulation (LBSL): *DARS2*
  - Pontoerebellar hypoplasia (PCH) type 6: *RARS2*
  - Leigh syndrome with specific lesions affecting the mamillothalamic tracts, substantia nigra, medial lemniscus, medial longitudinal fasciculus, spinothalamic tracts and cerebellum: *NDUFAF2*
- *^{1}H-MRS (spectroscopy)* of brain may reveal lactate accumulation.
- *Cranial CT* may reveal symmetrical hypodensities, or calcification e.g. in basal ganglia.

Open muscle biopsy (see also page 38)
This is usually the most important diagnostic investigation. If possible clinically affected tissue should be investigated. An open muscle biopsy, taken deep to the fascia and providing at least 200 mg tissue, is optimal to provide sufficient material for histology/histochemistry (+/– electron microscopy), spectrophotometric assay of respiratory chain enzymes, and molecular genetic investigation of mtDNA. The procedure should only be carried out in a specialised mitochondrial centre for optimal results. Specialist anaesthetic input is advisable. Some analyses (e.g. polarography and assay of complex V) can only be performed on fresh muscle, but these tests are not routinely performed in most mitochondrial diagnostic centres. Parts of the tissue samples should be treated as follows:
- Freeze in liquid nitrogen, store at –70°C:
  - Enzyme histochemistry (cytochrome C oxidase, SDH, ATPase)
  - Immunohistochemistry (antibodies against respiratory chain polypeptides)
  - Enzyme studies (see below)
  - Molecular genetic studies
- Fix for electron microscopy (mitochondrial number and morphology; abnormal mitochondria in general are a relatively non-specific finding)
- Immediate transfer of fresh tissue to mitochondrial lab for isolation and analysis of native mitochondria (e.g. measurement of oxidation of ^{14}C-labeled substrates or polarographic measurement of O_2 uptake)

Histochemical appearance
Typical abnormalities (common in adult mitochondrial disease, infrequent in children):
- Ragged red fibres (RRF, seen in modified Gomori trichrome stain) or ragged blue fibres (in combined COX/SDH stain); equivalent to SDH-positive fibres in SDH stain
- COX-negative fibres or strongly reduced overall COX staining (*caution*: technical problems – advisable to stain control at same time)
These findings all suggest an mtDNA mutation, although some mtDNA mutations (e.g. in complex I subunits) may not be associated with RRF. In addition, RRF may be observed in MDDS or in disorders of coenzyme Q_{10} biosynthesis. The absence of histopathological findings does not rule out a mitochondriopathy, while pathological findings may be of a secondary nature.

Ultrastructural appearance
Abnormalities of mitochondrial number and/or morphology in general are a relatively non-specific finding.

Biochemical analysis of PDHC deficiency and the respiratory chain

Most mitochondrial specialist laboratories perform spectrophotometric assays of complexes I to IV in frozen muscle homogenates. PDHC measurement should be routinely included in the diagnostic spectrum. Defects of the respiratory chain are identified in ~20% of cases with suspected mitochondrial disorders. The proportion is slightly higher in children, and lower in adults. Normal RC enzyme activities make a mitochondrial disorder less likely, but do not exclude it. Normal RC enzyme activities have been reported in many patients with mtDNA mutations, and in some patients with nuclear gene defects known to affect mitochondrial function, e.g. some cases with RARS2 mutations (a disorder of mitochondrial translation). It is also important to recognise that biochemical defects may be tissue-specific, e.g. confined to liver or heart. The most commonly identified defects (% of all identified enzyme defects) are:

• PDHC deficiency (~15%)
• Isolated complex I deficiency (~25–30%)
• Isolated complex IV deficiency (~25%)
• Multiple respiratory chain defects (~25–30%)

Isolated deficiencies of complex II or complex III appear to be rare. Deficiency of complex V is probably underdiagnosed, because some assays need to be performed on fresh tissue, and this service is not offered in most centres.

Liver biopsy

Histology in mitochondrial liver disease usually shows steatosis, often accompanied by fibrosis, cholestasis and loss of hepatocytes; COX staining may reveal reduced or patchy staining, e.g. in hepatocerebral MDDS.

Molecular genetics

• *Screen for common mtDNA deletions and point mutations*; consider whole mitochondrial genome sequence analysis. mtDNA mutations may be sporadic or maternally inherited. There may be a history of similar or disparate problems in maternal relatives, e.g. MELAS and MIDD are caused by same mtDNA mutation m.3243A>G in *MT-TL1*.
• *Quantitation of mtDNA* (in muscle or liver) if MDDS suspected
• *Mutation studies in nuclear genes* as indicated

Very few nuclear gene tests are available on a diagnostic basis at present, but this is likely to change. Nuclear gene defects causing mitochondrial disease show Mendelian (mostly aut. rec.) inheritance. A rapidly increasing number of nuclear genes is being reported to cause mitochondrial disease: already >80 genes are known, and these are listed below with the associated biochemical defect. The advent of next generation sequencing techniques will likely cause a steep increase in the number of nuclear genes known to cause mitochondrial disease.

Treatment

Currently no curative treatments exist for the overwhelming majority of mitochondrial disorders. Supportive treatments are the mainstay of therapy for these patients, and should be tailored to the individual's needs.

Potentially treatable disorders

• *Disorders of coenzyme Q_{10} biosynthesis*: high doses of coenzyme Q_{10} (30 mg/kg/day in children; total dose 1–4 g/day in adults)
• *Riboflavin-responsive complex I deficiency* (caused by *ACAD9* mutations): riboflavin (100–400 mg/day) (should be tried in all patients with isolated complex I deficiency)
• *PDHC deficiency* see *page 97*

General measures

A multidisciplinary team is required to provide supportive care for patients with mitochondrial disease.

- *Ensure adequate intake of energy, fluids and electrolytes*; avoid fasting
- *Exercise* – aerobic exercise should be encouraged
- *Avoid/treat conditions with high energy consumption*:
  - Treat fever efficiently
  - Treat seizures/epilepsy efficiently, avoid valproate
- *Treat acidosis* – sodium bicarbonate; THAM buffer if sodium is high; consider dialysis if necessary; dichloroacetate (inhibits PDH kinase, maintaining the PDH enzyme in an active state) may lower lactate levels but doubtful clinical value and risk of serious adverse effects (peripheral neuropathy)
- *Avoid drugs that may inhibit the respiratory chain or exaggerate symptoms* – e.g. valproate, barbiturates tetracyclines, chloramphenicol, aminoglycosides, propofol)
- *Anticonvulsants* – may need multiple drugs to control difficult seizures; avoid valproate
- *Hormonal replacement* – thyroxine, pancreatic enzyme supplements (eg Creon, Pancrex V), insulin, mineralo- and glucocorticoid replacement, growth hormone if deficiency detected
- *Blood transfusions* – for sideroblastic anaemia in Pearson syndrome
- *Hearing aids/cochlear implants* – depending on severity of hearing loss
- *Surgery for ptosis/PEO* – preferably by ophthalmologist experienced in mitochondrial disease
- *Cardiac pacing/transplantation* – regular monitoring for conduction defects and cardiomyopathy by specialist cardiologist, and appropriate intervention as indicated
- *Renal disease* – high dose electrolyte supplements may be needed for severe tubulopathy; dialysis/transplantation should be considered in end-stage renal failure

Trial of vitamins and cofactors to support mitochondrial function

- *Coenzyme Q_{10}*: 5–15 mg/kg/day (may need higher doses in primary coenzyme Q_{10} biosynthesis defects – see above)
- *Biotin*: 10–20 mg/day in suspected biotinidase deficiency
- *Thiamine (B_1)*: 150–300 mg/day in suspected PDH deficiency
- *Riboflavin (B_2)*: 100–400 mg/day especially in complex I deficiency

There is insufficient evidence that other vitamins or cofactors are helpful.

Experimental therapies

- *KSS* – folinic acid for cerebral folate (5MTHF) deficiency
- *LHON* – idebenone may protect vision if started soon after onset of visual loss in first eye
- *MELAS* – arginine therapy may be helpful to reduce number of stroke-like episodes; some evidence that i.v. treatment within 6 hours after onset of attacks ameliorates symptoms (keep Arg > 100 μmol/l)
- *MNGIE* – stem cell transplantation may be effective, but currently there is a high mortality associated with this treatment in MNGIE (~50%); earlier treatment may lead to an improved outcome
- *DGUOK* (if isolated hepatopathy) – liver transplantation

Reproductive options in mtDNA disorders

Risk to offspring possible in females; degree depends on type of mutation and tissue distribution/heteroplasmy. IVF with donor oocyte reduces recurrence risk to background levels. Prenatal diagnosis (PND) is problematic owing to heteroplasmy. Pre-implantation diagnosis (PGD) may be possible in extremely selected cases in some countries.

Leigh syndrome: Subacute necrotising encephalomyelopathy

Clinical:	Developmental delay/stepwise regression, growth retardation, hypotonia, ataxia, py-ramidal signs, symptoms/signs related to basal ganglia/brainstem dysfunction (dysto-nia, strabismus, nystagmus, optic atrophy, swallowing difficulties, vomiting); acute deterioration may occur after intercurrent infections
Onset:	Usually in infancy or early childhood; also late-onset forms
MRI:	Symmetric T2 hyperintensity of basal ganglia and brain stem, may be fluctuating (CT: bilateral fluctuating symmetrical hypodensities)
Pathol.:	Spongiform lesions with vacuolation of neuropil and relative preservation of neurons, associated with demyelination, gliosis, and capillary proliferation, bilaterally/symmet-rically especially in brainstem and basal ganglia
Genetics:	*Mitochondrial*: m.8993T>G/C (*MT-ATP6*); other mtDNA mutations *Aut. rec.*: *SURF1* (25–50% of Leigh + COX deficiency); *SDHA*, mutations in complex I subunit and assembly factor genes *X-chrom.*: *PDHA1*

Mitochondrial DNA depletion syndromes

Normal or elevated respiratory chain complex II in combination with reduced complexes I, III and IV indicate mtDNA depletion because all subunits of complex II are encoded by nuclear DNA. A reduced mtDNA copy number in muscle or liver is a diagnostic hallmark for disorders affecting mitochondrial DNA replication. All genes causing mtDNA depletion are nuclear, and so far all disorders follow aut. rec. inheritance. Onset of symptoms may range from the neonatal period to mid-childhood.

- *Hepatocerebral disease*: neonatal hypoglycaemia, liver dysfunction/failure (may mimick neo-natal haemochromatosis); global developmental delay, seizures, myoclonus, encephalopathy; infection-associated deterioration; overlap with Alpers (see below); *genes*: polymerase gamma catalytic subunit (*POLG*), deoxyguanosine kinase (*DGUOK*), twinkle protein (*C10ORF2*), *MPV17*
- *Navajo neurohepatopathy*: hepatopathy, peripheral neuropathy (Charcot joints), corneal anaes-thesia/scarring, leukoencephalopathy; *MPV17* gene
- *Progressive myopathy* presenting in infancy to mid-childhood (can mimic spinal muscular at-rophy): thimidine kinase 2; *TK2* gene
- *Encephalomyopathy* with Leigh-like lesions ± deafness and mild methylmalonic aciduria; *SUCLA2*, *SUCLG1* genes
- *Cerebrorenal disease*, encephalomyopathy + renal disesease; *RRM2B* gene

Alpers syndrome

Clinical:	*Progressive neuronal degeneration of childhood* (*PNDC*): intractable seizures (some-times epilepsia partialis continua) and liver involvement (latter may be triggered by sodium valproate)
Onset:	Early childhood (but can be later)
Pathol.:	*Brain, macroscopy*: patchy thinning and discolouration, with predilection for striate cortex (cerebral cortex variably involved) *Microscopy*: spongiosis, neuronal loss, and astrocytosis, which progresses down through the cortical layers; calcarine cortex is usually most affected (but all areas may be affected)
Genetics:	Aut. rec.; mostly *POLG* (frequent mutation p.A467T), rarely *C10ORF2*

MELAS syndrome

Clinical: Mitochondrial encephalomyopathy, lactic acidosis, stroke-like episodes: myopathy with ragged red fibres (RRF); migraine, vomiting, seizures (focal/generalised), hemiparesis, hemianopsia, cortical blindness, aphasia, progressive external opthalmoplegia (PEO), sensorineural hearing loss, dementia; diabetes mellitus, cardiomyopathy, short stature, renal disease. Milder affected patients in families due to heteroplasmy and heterogeneous tissue distribution.

Onset: 5–15 yrs

Genetics: *mtDNA mutations*: 80% m.3243A>G (*MT-TL1*) mostly maternally inherited, heterogeneous clinical presentations, most commonly MIDD (see next table); other mutations (e.g. *MT-ND5*) in most other cases, sporadic or mat. inherited; occasionally *POLG* mutations (aut. rec.)

Leber's hereditary optic neuropathy

Clinical: Subacute painless visual loss; sequentially affects both eyes; often associated with minor (occasionally major) neurological symptoms; males>females 4:1

Onset: 12–30 yrs

Genetics: *mtDNA mutations*: m.11778G>A (MT-ND4), m.3460G>A (MT-ND1), m.14484T>C (MT-ND6), others; usually homoplasmic; maternally inherited, variable penetrance (blindness in mutation carriers: males 50%, females 10%)

Progressive external opthalmoplegia (PEO)

Clinical: Ptosis (bilateral), limited peripheral vision due to limted eye movement; additional features may include proximal limb weakness, pharyngeal weakness, tremor, ataxia, depression, peripheral neuropathy, sensorineural hearing loss (SNHL), cataracts, endocrine dysfunction; feature of several mitochondrial syndromes

Onset: Early adulthood (20–30 yrs), occasionally childhood or late adulthood

Genetics: *Single mtDNA deletions* (50%, confined to skeletal muscle; sporadic, very low risk to offspring in females)
           Nuclear gene mutations: *POLG*, *POLG2*, *C10ORF2*, *SLC25A4*, *RRM2B* (aut. dom. = ADPEO); *POLG*, *RRM2B* (aut. rec. = ARPEO)

Diagn.:   mtDNA deletion analysis in muscle biopsy. Identification of multiple mtDNA deletions or mtDNA depletion indicate a primary nuclear gene disorder.

Kearns-Sayre syndrome (KSS)

Clinical: *Diagnostic triad*: (1) onset <age 20 yrs, (2) PEO, (3) pigmentary retinopathy
           In addition at least one of (a) cardiac conduction block, (b) cerebellar ataxia, (c) CSF protein >0.1 g/l
           Other features: growth failure; deafness; endocrine deficiencies

Onset: Childhood (<20 yrs)

Genetics: *Large mtDNA deletions* ± *duplications* (90%); occasionally aut. rec. (e.g. *RRM2B*)

Diagn.:   mtDNA deletion analysis in blood (usually present in childhood) or urine; if mtDNA analysis in blood and urine negative but clinical suspicion persists, proceed to muscle biopsy

Pearson syndrome

Clinical: *Marrow pancreas syndrome:* anaemia/pancytopenia, exocrine pancreatic dysfunction, liver dysfunction, failure to thrive, high mortality in childhood; survivors may later go on to develop KSS
Onset: Infancy
Genetics: Large mtDNA deletions ± duplications (sporadic)
Diagn.:   mtDNA deletion analysis in blood (usually present) or urine; if mtDNA analysis in blood and urine negative but clinical suspicion persists, proceed to muscle biopsy

Mitochondrial neuro-gastro-intestinal encephalopathy (MNGIE)

Clinical: Demyelinating neuropathy (can mimic chronic inflammatory demyelinating polyneuropathy, CIDP), episodes of intestinal pseudo-obstruction, myopathy, PEO, leukoencephalopathy
Onset: 5–15 yrs
Genetics: *TYMP* mutations (aut. rec.)
Diagn.:   Increased thymidine and deoxyuridine levels in plasma and urine; thymidine phosphorylase deficiency (platelets or leukocytes); multiple mtDNA deletions and/or depletion in muscle biopsy
Therapy: Allogeneic stem cell transplantation may be curative if performed early in disease course

Reversible mitochondrial disease

• *Infantile reversible myopathy*: early-onset severe muscle weakness, hypotonia, lactic acidosis; may need assisted ventilation; spontaneous improvement from 5–20 mths; multiple respiratory chain deficiencies in initial biopsies, later normal; mild residual myopathy; associated with homoplasmic mtDNA mutation m.14674T>C (*MT-TE*), variable penetrance
• *Reversible liver disease*: acute liver failure and lactic acidosis in infancy, may be fatal; if survival: improvement from 2–3 wks, normal liver function from 3–4 mths, normal development; aut. rec. inheritance, *TRMU* gene

Other mitochondrial disorders caused by mutations in mtDNA

Syndrome	Clinical features	Onset (age)	Genetic defect
MERRF	Myoclonic epilepsy with RRF; encephalomyopathy, neuropathy, progressive dementia, occasionally multiple symmetrical lipomatosis	5–15 yrs	m.8344G>A (*MT-TK*); other mtDNA mutations
NARP	Neuropathy, ataxia, retinitis pigmentosa	5–30 yrs	m.8993T>G/C (*MT-ATP6*) (mat. inherited)
MIDD	Maternally inherited diabetes and deafness	20–30 yrs	m.3243A>G (MT-TL1)

Other mitochondrial disorders caused by mutations in nuclear DNA

Syndrome	Clinical features	Onset (age)	Genetic defect
Barth	Cardiomyopathy, cyclical neutropenia, myopathy, short stature; see *page 63*	Neonate/ infancy	*TAZ* (X-linked)
DCMA	Dilated cardiomyopathy with ataxia, similar to Barth but aut. rec.		*DNAJC19* (aut. rec.)
Sengers	Congenital cataract, hypertrophic cardio-myopathy, myopathy, lactic acidosis	Neonate	Unknown
Ethylmalonic encephalo-pathy	Developmental delay, acrocyanosis, petechi-ae, diarrhoea; see *page 64*	Neonate/ infancy	*ETHE1* (aut. rec.)
GRACILE	Growth retardation, aminoaciduria, cholesta-sis, iron overload, lactic acidosis and early death; allelic with *Björnstad syndrome* = congenital SNHL, pili torti	Neonate/ infancy	*BCS1L* (aut. rec.)
MLASA	Myopathy, lactic acidosis, sideroblastic anaemia	Infancy–childhood	*PUS1, YARS2* (aut. rec.)
Mohr-Tranebjaerg	Deafness dystonia syndrome: SNHL, pro-gressive visual disability leading to cortical blindness, dystonia, fractures, mental defi-ciency, dementia	3–5 yrs	*TIMM8A* (X-linked)
Optic atro-phy type 1 (Kjer-type)	Bilateral symmetrical optic atrophy; neuro-logical manifestations in ~20% of cases: SNHL, ataxia, myopathy, neuropathy, PEO	4–6 yrs 20–30 yrs	*OPA1* (aut. dom.)
Wolfram	DIDMOAD; bladder instability, ataxia, peripheral neuropathy, dementia, psychiatric disorders, seizures	3–40 yrs (by teens in most cases)	*WFS1* (aut. rec.)
SANDO	Sensory ataxia, neuropathy, dysarthria, ophthalmoplegia: phenotype also includes myopathy, seizures, migraine, SNHL; over-lap with SCAE and MIRAS	20–30 yrs	*POLG* (aut. rec.)

DIDMOAD = Diabetes insipidus, diabetes mellitus, optic atrophy, deafness, MIRAS = mitochon-drial recessive ataxia syndrome, PEO = progressive external ophthalmoplegia, SCAE = spino-cerebellar ataxia with epilepsy, SNHL = sensineural hearing loss

Isolated complex I deficiency
- *Subunit mutations* – *MT-ND1–6*, *MT-ND4L*, mtDNA deletions and tRNA point mutations (spo-radic or mat inherit), *NDUFS1–4*, *NDUFS6–8*, *NDUFV1–2*, *NDUFA2*, *NDUFA11* (all aut. rec.), *NDUFA1* (X-linked)
- *Assembly factor mutations* – *NDUFAF1–4*, *C20ORF7*, *C8ORF38*, *FOXRED1*, *NUBPL*, *ACAD9* (all aut. rec.)

Isolated complex II deficiency
- *Subunit mutations – SDHA* (aut. rec. Leigh syndrome); *SDHB-D* (aut. dom. paraganglioneuromas and phaeochromocytomas)
- Assembly factor mutations – *SDHAF1* (aut. rec.), *SDHAF2* (aut. dom.)

Isolated complex III deficiency
- *Subunit mutations – MT-CYB1* (mtDNA), *UQCRB, UQCRQ* (aut. rec.)
- *Assembly factor mutations – BCS1, HCCS, TTC19* (aut. rec.)

Isolated complex IV deficiency
- *Subunit mutations – MT-CO1–3* (mtDNA), *COX4I2, COX6B1* (aut. rec.)
- *Assembly factor mutations – SURF1, COX10, COX15, SCO1, SCO2, LRPPRC, FASTKD2, TACO1* (all aut. rec.)

Isolated complex V deficiency
- *Subunit mutations – MT-ATP6,8* (mtDNA), *ATP5E* (aut. rec.)
- *Assembly factor mutations – ATPAF2, TMEM70* (aut. rec.)

Multiple respiratory chain defects
- *Disorders of mtDNA maintenance* usually cause deficiency of complexes I, III and IV (and V where measured), but may have isolated defects of complex I or complex IV in early disease stages; RC assays are frequently normal in adults with PEO caused by mtDNA replication defects; genes: see mtDNA depletion syndromes and PEO (multiple mtDNA deletions)
- *Disorders of mitochondrial translation* [deficiency of any combination of complexes I, III, IV and V] – mtDNA deletions or point mutations in tRNA genes (mtDNA); *PUS1, MRPS16, MRPS22, GFM1, TSFM, TUFM, DARS2, RARS2, SARS2, YARS2, TRMU, C12ORF65, MTPAP, SPG7, AFG3L2* (all aut. rec.)
- *Disorders of coenzyme Q_{10} biosynthesis* cause deficiency of complexes I + III or II + III when assayed together, but normal activities of complexes I, II + III when assayed separately (linked assays are dependent on endogenous coenzyme Q_{10}) – *COQ2, PDSS1, PDSS2, ADCK3, COQ9* (aut. rec.)
- *Disorders of mitochondrial import: SLC25A3, SLC25A12, SLC25A19, SLC25A38, DNAJC19* (aut. rec.), *TIMM8A* (X-linked)
- *Disorders of mitochondrial dynamics* [NB respiratory chain biochemistry may be normal in muscle in these disorders] – *MFN2, OPA1* (aut. dom.), *DLP1, AIFM1* (X-linked)

Disorders of transporters across the mitochondrial membrane
Genes coding for mitochondrial membrane solute carriers are denoted SLC25.
- *Glutamate carrier (SLC25A22 gene):* neonatal myoclonic epilepsy
- *ADP/ATP carrier (SLC25A4 gene):* aut. dom. progressive external ophthalmoplegia, exercise intolerance
- *Phosphate carrier (SLC25A3 gene):* hypotonia, cardiomyopathy, lactic acidosis
- *Carnitine acylcarnitine carrier (SLC25A20 gene)* (see *page 92*)
- *Ornithine/citruline carrier (SLC25A15 gene):* HHH syndrome (see *page 59*)
- *Asparate glutamate carrier (SLC25A13 gene):* citrin deficiency (see *page 60*)
- *Thiamine-PP carrier (SLC25A19 gene):* Amish type microcephaly (see *page 161*)

Disorders of creatine biosynthesis

Biochemistry
Creatine is synthesised in a two-step process involving *arginine:glycine amidinotransferase* (AGAT) and *guanidinoacetate methyltransferase* (GAMT); S-adenosylmethionine (SAM) serves as methyl donor. A *creatine transporter* (CRTR) is required for creatine uptake into brain and muscle.

The creatine/creatine-phosphate system serves as a cytosolic storage buffer of chemical energy in brain and muscle.

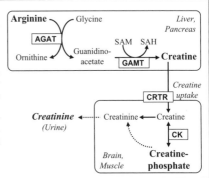

Disorders of creatine biosynthesis or transport cause *intellectual disability, speech impairment and epilepsy* due to cerebral creatine deficiency. Low creatine concentrations in the brain may be recognised by NMR spectroscopy (MRS); abnormal concentrations of creatine/creatinine and its precursor guanidinoacetate may be found in serum and urine.

Guanidinoacetate methyltransferase (GAMT) deficiency
Clinical: Intellectual disability, epilepsy; 80% behavioural disorders (incl. autistic behaviours, self-mutilation); 45% pyramidal/extrapyramidal findings
Diagn.: ↓ Creatine/creatinine (urine), ↑ guanidinoacetate (plasma, urine, CSF); ↓↓ creatine (MRS brain); (allopurinol test may be pathological); *GAMT* gene
Therapy: Creatine 400 mg/kg/day, 3–6 doses; reduction of accumulating guanidino acetic acid (GAA) by ornithine supplementation 100–800 mg/kg/day (may be combined with arginine restriction 15–25 mg/kg/day)

Arginine:glycine amidinotransferase (AGAT) deficiency
Clinical: Rare; intellectual disability
Diagn.: ↓ Guanidinoacetate (plasma, urine), n–↓ creatine/creatinine (urine); ↓↓ creatine (MRS brain); *GATM* gene
Therapy: Creatine 300–400 mg/kg/day

Creatine transporter deficiency
May be found in up to 2% of males with non-syndromic X-linked intellectual disability with or without epilepsy.
Clinical: *Males*: variable from mild intellectual disability and speech delay to severe intellectual disability, seizures, and behavioural disorder
Females: 50% learning and behavioural problems
Genetics: X-chromosomal; *SLC6A8* gene
Diagn.: ↑ Creatine/creatinine ratio (diagnostic), normal guanidinoacetate (urine); ↓↓ creatine (MRS brain)
Therapy: No effective therapy

Purine and pyrimidine metabolism

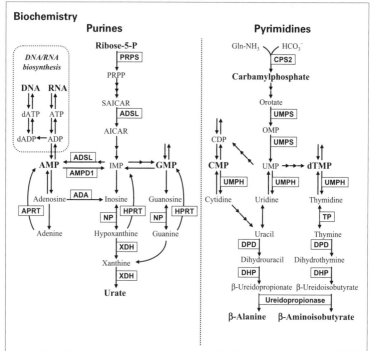

Purine biosynthesis involves a complex pathway resulting in inosine monophosphate (IMP) which is converted into adenosine or guanosine monophosphate (AMP, GMP). Purines are catabolised via hypoxanthine and xanthine to uric acid.

Pyrimidine biosynthesis starts with carbamylphosphate (synthesised by cytosolic carbamyl-phosphate synthase II [CPS2] – for CPS1 see *page 57*) and, via orotic acid (see also *page 36*), leads to uridine monophopsphate (UMP) and subsequently cytidine or thymidine compounds. DNA and RNA biosynthesis is shown on the example of AMP. For enzyme abbreviations see text.

Clinical features
- Renal manifestations: recurrent urinary tract infections, nephrolithiasis, renal failure
- Neurological manifestations: psychomotor retardation, epilepsy, spasticity, dystonia, ataxia, autism, self-mutilation, deafness
- Arthritis
- Small stature
- Muscle cramps and muscle wasting
- Anaemia
- Immunodeficiency with recurrent infections

mtDNA depletion syndromes
Deficiencies of several enzymes in purine/pyrimidine metabolism cause mtDNA depletion (see *page 106*). These include:
- Deoxyguanosine kinase deficiency (*DGUOK* gene)
- Mitochondrial ribonucleotide reductase subunit 2 deficiency (*RRM2B* gene)
- Thymidine phosphorylase deficiency (*TK2* gene)

Investigations
- Uric acid in serum, total uric acid in 24-hr urine
- Uric acid per creatinine in morning urine (mol/mol = $0.67 \times$ mg/mg):

Uric acid	Neonates	1st yr	Age 2–5	Age 6–14	Adults
mol/mol creatinine	0.2–3	0.2–2	0.2–1.5	0.2–1	0.15–0.6

  - Elevated: PRPS superactivity, Lesch-Nyhan syndrome, familial juvenile hyperuricaemic nephropathy
  - Decreased: NP deficiency, xanthinuria, nucleotidase hyperactivity
- Urine crystals
- Purines and pyrimidines in urine by HPLC (see *page 37*)
  - 24-hr urine, alternatively morning urine (purine and pyrimidine excretion is affected by the diet and may vary considerably during the day)
  - Avoid methylxanthines (coffee, black tea, cocoa, liquorice) one day before and during urine collection
  - Exclude renal tract infection
  - For the diagnosis of neurological disease: freeze urine immediately, ship on dry ice (unstable marker metabolites in adenylosuccinase deficiency)

Disorders of purine metabolism

Phosphoribosyl pyrophosphate synthetase (PRPS) superactivity
Clinical: Hyperuricaemia → nephrolithiasis, gout, sensorineural deafness
Manif.: Young men (in children: deafness, intellectual disability, ataxia, hypotonia, dysmorphism)
Bioch.: Overproduction of IMP; *PRPS1* gene, X-chromosomal
Diagn.: ↑ Uric acid, ↑ hypoxanthine
Therapy: Diet (purine-restricted); alkalise urine, plentiful fluids; allopurinol (2–)10–20 mg/kg/day (beware of xanthine stones – monitor xanthine and oxypurinol)
Note: Hypomorphic (loss of function) mutations in *PRPS1* cause Arts syndrome (neuropathy, infections, optic atrophy, deafness), X-linked Charcot-Marie-Tooth disease-5 (*CMTX5*), and X-linked nonsyndromic sensorineural deafness (*DFN2*).

Adenylosuccinate lyase (ADSL) deficiency

Clinical: Severe psychomotor retardation, epilepsy, autism, ataxia, sometimes growth retardation

Manif.: Neonates, infants

Bioch.: Disorder of purine (IMP) and specifically AMP biosynthesis; *ADSL* gene

Diagn.: Positive Bratton-Marshal test; ↑ Succinyladenosine, ↑ SAICA riboside; AA after acid hydrolysis: ↑ Asp, Gly

5-Amino-4-imidazolecarboxamide ribsosiduria (AICAR-uria)

Clinical: Severe psychomotor retardation, blindness, epilepsy, dysmorphic features

Manif.: Neonates, infants

Enzyme: AICAR formyltransferase/IMP cyclohydrolase; *ATIC* gene

Bioch.: Disorder of purine biosynthesis (IMP)

Diagn.: Positive Bratton-Marshal test; ↑ AICA riboside in erythrocytes

Myoadenylate deaminase (muscle AMP deaminase, AMPD1) deficiency

Clinical: Exercise: rapid fatigue, muscle cramps

Manif.: From childhood (often few or no symptoms)

Diagn.: ↑ CK; *AMPD1* gene

Therapy: Consider ribose 2–60 g/day

Adenosine deaminase (ADA) deficiency

Clinical: Severe combined immunodeficiency (SCID); diarrhoea, failure to thrive; progressive neurological symptoms (spasticity, movement disorder)

Manif.: Neonatal (rarely up to school age)

Bioch.: Inhibition of ribonucleotide reductase by adenosine; *ADA* gene

Diagn.: Blood count: lymphopenia; hypogammaglobulinaemia; ↑ adenosine

Therapy: Bone marrow transplantation, enzyme replacement (expensive), gene therapy

Purine nucleoside phosphorylase (NP) deficiency

Clinical: Cellular immunodeficiency; immunohaemolytic anaemia, progressive neurological symptoms (spasticity, movement disorder, retardation) more frequent than in ADA deficiency

Manif.: 1–6 yrs, rarely later

Diagn.: ↓ Uric acid, ↑ inosine, guanosine (deficient breakdown); *PNP* gene

Therapy: Bone marrow transplantation

Xanthinuria

Clinical: Haematuria, nephrolithiasis (xanthine = radiolucent), renal failure, arthropathy, myopathy, often asymptomatic (> 50% of homozygotes)

Manif.: From early childhood

Enzyme: Xanthine oxidase = xanthine dehydrogenase; *XDH* gene

Var.: *Molybdenum cofactor deficiency*: also sulphite oxidase deficiency (see *page 71*)
Xanthinuria type II: combined deficiency of xanthine dehydrogenase and aldehyde oxidase, gene unknown

Diagn.: ↓ Uric acid, ↑↑ xanthine, ↑ hypoxanthine

Therapy: Diet (purine-restricted), plentiful fluids, if residual activity: allopurinol

Familial juvenile hyperuricaemic nephropathy (HNFJ)

Clinical: Gout, early renal failure
Manifest.: From puberty
Genes: *UMOD* (uromodulin, HNFJ type I) or *REN* (rennin, HNFJ type II)
Diagn.:   Hyperuricaemia, ↓ renal uric acid excretion; positive family history

Lesch-Nyhan syndrome

Clinical: Motor retardation, muscular hypotonia, dystonia, choreoathetosis, spasticity, epilep-
           sy, self-mutilation; uric acid stones (radiolucent) → renal failure; gout
Manif.:   From 3–4 mths, progressive deterioration
Enzyme: Hypoxanthine:guanine phosphoribosyltransferase, *HPRT* gene, X-linked!
Bioch.:   Deficient regeneration of IMP (from hypoxanthine) and GMP (from guanine)
Var.:   Mild forms: gout, occasionally few neurological symptoms
Diagn.:   ↑↑ Uric acid (morning urine: ↑ uric acid per creatinine), ↑ hypoxanthine
Therapy: Diet (purine-restricted), plentiful fluids, high dose allopurinol; symptomatic (neuro-
           logical complications)

Adenine phosphoribosyltransferase (APRT) deficiency

Clinical: Nephrolithiasis (2,8-dihydroxyadenine) → renal failure
Manif.:   All age groups (neonatal to old age) may be asymptomatic
Diagn.:   ↑ Adenine, 2,8-dihydroxyadenine (adenine metabolite, produced by XDH); *APRT*
           gene
Therapy: Diet (purine-restricted), plentiful fluids, allopurinol; do not alkalise urine

Disorders of pyrimidine metabolism

Hereditary orotic aciduria

Clinical: Megaloblastic anaemia, not responding to treatment → failure to thrive, retardation
Manif.:   Neonate, infant
Enzyme: Uridine-monophosphate synthase; *UMPS* gene
Bioch.:   Pyrimidine deficiency
Diagn.:   ↑↑ Orotic acid
Therapy: Uridine (25–)100–150 mg/kg/day (monitor therapy: urinary orotic acid)

Pyrimidine 5′-nucleotidase deficiency

Clinical: Chronic haemolytic anaemia (basophilic stippling)
Enzyme: Uridine monophosphate hydrolase (UMPH); *NT5C* gene
Diagn.:   Erythrocyte analysis (↑ glutathione; nucleotide profile)
DD: Chronic lead intoxication (inhibitor of UMPH)
Progn.:   Relatively good; transfusions rarely necessary

Dihydropyrimidine dehydrogenase (DPD) deficiency
Clinical: Frequently asymptomatic, sometimes intellectual disability, epilepsy, microcephaly, failure to thrive; severe (occasionally fatal) 5-fluorouracil toxicity in asymptomatic patients and heterozygotes
Diagn.:   ↑ Uracil, thymine (insufficient degradation); *DPYD* gene

Dihydropyrimidinase (DHP) deficiency
Clinical: Similar to DPD deficiency, may be asymptomatic
Diagn.:   ↑ Dihydrouracil, dihydrothymine (OA urine), ↑ uracil, thymine; *DPYS* gene

Ureidopropionase deficiency
Clinical: Similar to DPD deficiency, dystonia
Diagn.:   n–↑ Dihydrouracil, dihydrothymine (OA urine), n–↑ uracil, thymine; ↑ ureido-propionate, β-alanine (arises during analysis), ureidoisobutyrate; *UPB1* gene

Other disorders of nucleotide metabolism

- *Nucleotidase hyperactivity*: intellectual disability, seizures, ataxia, behavioural abnormalities; diagn.: ↓ (or low normal) uric acid/creatinine, otherwise normal results incl. purine and pyrimidine studies, gene unknown; ↑ nucleotidase activity (fibroblasts); therapy: uridine 50 mg/kg (up to 1,000 mg/kg)

Sterol metabolism

Disorders of sterol biosynthesis

Sterol synthesis defects present clinically as *multi-system disorders with dysmorphic features and variable skeletal dysplasies*; they should also be considered in cases of otherwise unexplained recurrent abortions and fetal dysmorphism. The biochemical diagnosis is not always straight-forward: Serum cholesterol is usually normal in all disorders except (sometimes) Smith-Lemli-Opitz syndrome (SLOS), and even specific sterol analysis may yield normal results. In these instances the diagnosis can be reached by mutation analysis or functional studies (fibroblasts cultured in sterol-free media). Pathogenesis appears to be related mostly to prenatal development in all disorders except mevalonate kinase deficiency and SLOS. Treatment with cholesterol is rarely warranted except in patients with hypocholesterolaemia and SLOS.

Biochemistry

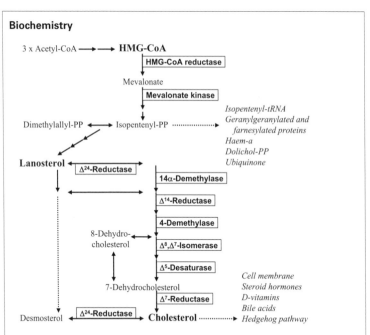

The first step of cholesterol biosynthesis is the cytosolic condensation of three acetyl-CoA to 3-hydroxy-3-methylglutaryl-(HMG-)CoA, which is then converted via mevalonic acid to activated isoprenoids. Further modification and condensation produces lanosterol, the first sterol and precursor of cholesterol.

Mevalonic aciduria, hyper-IgD syndrome

Clinical: *Mevalonic aciduria*: dysmorphism, dystrophy, progressive ataxia due to cerebellar atrophy, psychomotor retardation, retinitis pigmentosa, recurrent crises with fever, skin
rash, lymphadenopathy, hepatosplenomegaly
Hyper-IgD syndrome: recurrent febrile attacks

Enzyme: Mevalonate kinase; *MVK* gene

Bioch.: Disorder of the biosynthesis of cholesterol and isoprenoids

Diagn.: OA (urine): ($\uparrow$) Mevalonic acid, mevalonolactone (typically > 500 mmol/mol creatinine in mevalonic aciduria, < 100 mmol/mol creatine in hyper-IgD syndrome); $\uparrow$ leukotrienes, prostanoids (urine); serum: $\uparrow$ CK, IgD, transaminases, n–$\downarrow$ cholesterol

Therapy: Intermittent high-dose prednisone or IL-1 receptor antagonist anakinra; substitution
with ubiquinone, vit. E and C; allogenic bone marrow transplantation in case of severe, life-threatening inflammatory attacks

Desmosterolosis

Clinical: Facial dysmorphism, cleft palate, multiple malformations, ambiguous genitalia, short
limbs, osteosclerosis, psychomotor retardation

Enzyme: 3β-Hydroxysterol/desmosterol Δ^{24}-reductase); *DHCR24* gene

Bioch.: Disorder of the biosynthesis of cholesterol but not of isoprenoids

Diagn.: Sterols (plasma, fibroblasts): $\uparrow$ desmosterol

Antley-Bixler syndrome (Lanosterolosis)

Clinical: Craniofacial dysmorphism, cranyiosynostosis, radiohumeral synostosis, contractures;
genital anomalies (males + females)

Enzyme: Cytochrome P_{450} oxidoreductase, POR (donates electrons to all microsomal P_{450} enzymes, e.g. lanosterol 14α-demethylase = CYP51A1), *POR* gene

Diagn.: Sterols (plasma, fibroblasts): $\uparrow$ lanosterol, dihydrolanosterol

DD: Antley-Bixler syndrome may also be due to heterozygous *FGFR2* mutations (no genital anomalies, normal steroidogenesis)

3β-Hydroxysterol Δ^{14}-reductase

Two different proteins appear to be able to catalyse this reaction: the nuclear lamin B receptor
(*LBR* gene) and the product of the *TM7SF2* gene, also denoted as DHCR14. *LBR* mutations cause
a range of phenotypes from *Pelger-Huët anomaly* (abnormal granulocytes in heterozygotes) to
Greenberg dysplasia (hydrops, skeletal dysplasia, fragmented long bones, ectopic calcifications;
homozygous *LBR* mutations). Sterol anomalies ($\uparrow$ cholesta-8,14-diene-3-betaol) may be found in
Greenberg dysplasia, but symptoms may be due to deficient lamin B function, not abnormal steroidogenesis.

Sterol-C4-methyl oxidase deficiency

Clinical: Psoriasiform dermatitis, arthralgias, congenital cataracts, microcephaly, intellectual
disability

Diagn.: $\downarrow$ Cholesterol (serum); sterols (plasma, fibroblasts): $\uparrow$ 4-methylsterols; *SC4MOL* mutations

CHILD syndrome (X-linked dominant)

Clinical: *Females*: "congenital hemidysplasia with ichthyosiform nevus and limb defects": unilateral ichthyotic skin lesions with a sharp demarcation at the midline of the trunk, stippled epiphyses on the affected side
Males: null mutations lethal; hypomorphic mutations dysmorphic syndrome with intellectual disability, microcephaly, cortical malformation, thin habitus

Enzyme: 3β-Hydroxysterol 4-demethylase, *NSDHL* gene, X-chrom. (Xq28), heterozygous mutations, unilateral phenotype unexplained

Diagn.: Sterols (plasma, fibroblasts): ↑ 4-methylsterols

Therapy: Experimental: cholesterol 50–150 mg/kg in patients with hypocholesterolaemia or active skin disease

Chondrodysplasia punctata Conradi-Hünermann (X-linked, CDPX2)

Clinical: *Females*: rhizomelic short stature with asymmetric shortening of proximal limbs, stippled epiphyses, sectorial cataracts, ichthyosis, intellectual disability
Males: lethal

Enzyme: 3β-Hydroxysterol Δ^8,Δ^7-isomerase, *EBP* gene, X-chrom. (Xp11.2)

Diagn.: Sterols (plasma, fibroblasts): ↑ 8-Dehydrocholesterol, 8(9)-cholestenol

DD: See *page 144*; RCDP1

Therapy: Experimental: cholesterol 50–150 mg/kg in patients with hypocholesterolaemia or active skin disease

Lathosterolosis

Clinical: Severe malformations, overlapping the spectrum of Smith-Lemli-Opitz syndrome; lipid storage

Enzyme: 3β-Hydroxysterol Δ^5-desaturase; *SC5DL* gene

Diagn.: Sterols (plasma, fibroblasts): ↑ lathosterol

Therapy: Lipid storage might be aggravated by supplemental cholesterol

Smith-Lemli-Opitz syndrome

Clinical: *Malformations*: craniofacial dysmorphism (microcephaly, micrognathia, anteverted nostrils, ptosis); syndactyly of 2nd and 3rd toes (almost obligatory); renal, cardiac, gastrointestinal and mid-line malformations incl. holoprosencephaly, genital malformations in boys; (compensated) adrenal insufficiency may decompensate during illnes; *intellectual disability*, behavioural disturbances, feeding problems, failure to thrive; very variable severity ranging from intra-uterine death to normal life span

Enzyme: 3β-Hydroxysterol Δ^7-reductase; *DHCR7* gene

Bioch.: Defect of the last step of cholesterol biosynthesis

Diagn.: Sterols (plasma, fibroblasts): ↑ 7-Dehydrocholesterol (7-DHC) and 8-DHC; n–↓ cholesterol

Therapy: Cholesterol 50–100 mg/kg, higher in infants; simvastatin 0.5–1 mg/kg in 2 doses may be useful in mildly affected patients. In an acute illness, when enteral cholesterol supplementation cannot be continued, frozen plasma can be given as an emergency source of LDL cholesterol.

Disorders of bile acid synthesis

Biochemistry
Bile acids are synthesised from cholesterol in the liver. The first reaction (7α-hydroxylation) is rate-limiting; some steps involve peroxisomal β-oxidation. The two main bile acids, cholic and chenodesoxycholic acids, are activated to CoA esters, conjugated with either glycine or taurine to form bile salts and excreted into the bile. Bile acids are essential for lipid resorption in the gut, they regulate hepatic cholesterol synthesis (inhibition of HMG-CoA reductase) and are necessary for adequate bile production.

Bile acid synthesis defects with cholestasis and malabsorption

Clinical: Prolonged neonatal jaundice, steatorrhoea, treatment-resistant diarrhoea, rickets, haemorrhage, sometimes hepatosplenomegaly, pruritus

Enzymes: • 3β-Hydroxy-Δ^5-C_{27}-sterol dehydrogenase; *HSD3B7* gene (= PFIC type 4)
           • Δ^4-3-Oxosterol 5β-reductase; *AKR1D1* gene
           • Oxysterol 7α-hydroxylase; *CYP7B1* gene

Diagn.:   (n–)↑ Conjugated bilirubin, transaminases, AP, PTT; normal γGT; n–↓ calcium, n–↓ cholesterol; ↓ vit. E, D, K, A; ↑ specific bile acids (bile, plasma, urine)

DD: α-Methyl-acyl-CoA racemase deficiency (see *page 145*)
      Progressive familial intrahepatic cholestasis (PFIC): hepatobiliary transport deficiencies (different genes, aut. rec.) → jaundice, pruritus, growth retardation, hepato(spleno) megaly, cirrhosis; hyperbilirubinaemia (mixed); ↑ transaminases, ↑ AP; GGT usually normal; may require liver transplantation
      Byler disease = PFIC type I, *ATP8B1* gene

Therapy: Substitution of bile acids

Progn.:   Good except for oxysterol 7α-hydroxylase deficiency which may require liver transplantation

---

Cerebrotendinous xanthomatosis

Clinical: Self-limiting neonatal hepatitis; psychomotor retardation, treatment-resistant diarrhoea, cataract (specific type), later xanthomas (from 2nd decade); atherosclerosis, osteoporosis; progressive ataxia → dementia

Enzyme: Sterol 27-hydroxylase, *CYP27A1* gene

Bioch.:   Accumulation of cholestanol (and cholesterol) particularly in the nervous system

Diagn.:   (↑) Cholestanol, n–↑ cholesterol (plasma); ↑ specific bile alcohols (urine)

Therapy: Substitution of bile acids, statins

Other disorders of bile acid biosynthesis

• *Cholesterol 7α-hydroxylase deficiency* (*CYP7A1* gene): hypercholesterolaemia, hypertriglyceridaemia, gallstones
• *Bile acid amidation defect* (*BAAT* gene): cholestatic liver disease, rickets

Porphyrin and haem metabolism

Biochemistry

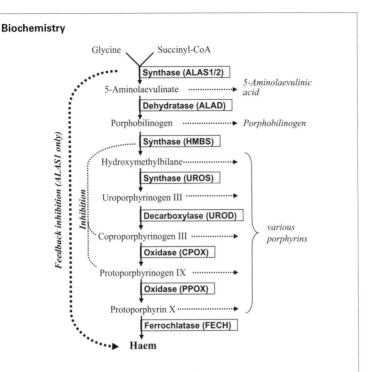

Biosynthesis of haem from glycine and succinyl-CoA involves eight enzymatic steps and takes place mainly in the bone marrow (80%) and liver (15%). The first enzyme, 5-amino-laevulinate synthase is coded by two genes, one erythroid-specific (ALAS2, X-chromosomal) and one ubiquitous (ALAS1). ALAS1 is the rate-limiting enzyme in hepatic haem production; it is controlled via negative feedback by intracellular haem. ALAS2 is actively induced for haem synthesis, its rate is limited by iron availability. Haem is metabolised to bilirubin and excreted via bile.

Porphyrias are often classified as hepatic or erythropoietic according to the organ in which haem precursors accumulate. However, a clinical classification is more useful for practical purposes. Depending on the accumulating metabolites, porphyrias present with *acute neuropathic symptoms* (5-aminolaevulinic acid, porphobilinogen) or *photosensitivity dermatoses* (porphyrins). Many porphyrias are inherited as aut. dom. traits.

Investigations

- Screening tests for porphobilinogen in urine (Hoesch test, Watson-Schwartz test) when acute hepatic porphyria is suspected
- Specific analyses (urine, faeces, erythrocytes; see *page 37*)

Acute neuropathic porphyrias

Clinical: Acute episodes of severe abdominal pain, limb pain, sympathetic overactivity (tachycardia, hypertension, tremor), vomiting, constipation, electrolyte imbalance, mental disturbance, development of peripheral neuropathy, weakness, seizures; lasting days to weeks

Pathogen.: Accumulation of highly neurotoxic 5-aminolaevulinic acid + porphobilinogen as a combined effect of upregulated hepatic haem biosynthesis and reduced capacity of porphobilinogen deaminase (or amnionlaevulate dehydratase)

Triggers: Various drugs (particularly cytochrome P_{450} enzyme inducers), hormones (progesterone), nutritional factors (low cellular glucose), smoking, alcohol, stress, ond others

Diagn.: ↑–↑↑ porphobilinogen, aminolaevulinic acid in urine (acute episodes, mostly normal in remission)

Therapy: *Acute*: intensive care monitoring, stop adverse drugs, analgesia (opiates, chlorpromazine) antiemetics (promazine), i.v. glucose (4–6 g/kg/day), haemin (3–4 mg/kg/day as short infusion over 4 days)
Long-term: avoid triggers

- *Acute intermittent porphyria*: hydroxymethylbilane synthase (*HMBS* gene) (previous name porphobilinogen deaminase), aut. dom., low penetrance (10–50%); manifestation age 20–40 yrs, ♀ > ♂ (2:1); common; diagn.: same as above, normal faecal porphyrins, enzyme studies (erythrocytes): 50% activity
- *Porphyria variegata*: protoporphyrinogen oxidase (*PPOX* gene), aut. dom.; 50% penetrance; bullous photodermatosis common, only symptom in 60% of patients; diagn.: same as above, ↑ faecal coproporphyrin + protoporphyrin
- *Hereditary coproporphyria*: coproporphyrinogen oxidase (*CPOX* gene), aut. dom.; photodermatosis rare (5%); diagn.: same as above; ↑ faecal coproporphyrin
- *Aminolaevulinate dehydratase porphyria* (porphobilinogen synthase, *ALAD* gene): aut. rec., rare; enzyme analysis in DBS possible

Porphyrias with erosive photodermatosis

Clinical: Sun-exposed skin: fragility, erosions (secondary infections), crusts, blisters; hypertrichosis, hyperpigmentation, scarring alopecia; liver dysfunction

Diagn.: Specific porphyrins in urine, faeces and blood

Therapy: Avoid exposure to sunlight (sunblock!); avoid alcohol, smoking, unsafe drugs
PCT: chloroquine (2 × 125 mg/wk); if iron overload: phlebotomy
CEP: transfusion, bone marrow transplantation

* *Porphyria cutanea tarda* (PCT, chronic hepatic porphyria): uroporphyrinogen-III decarboxylase (*UROD* gene), aut. dom., reduced penetrance; *sporadic PCT* (75% of cases): no *UROD* mutations, normal erythrocyte UROD activity, unclear pathogenesis; most common porphyria world-wide; adult onset
  Risk factors: alcohol, oestrogens, hepatitis C, genetic haemochromatosis
  Diagn.: ↑ uroporphyrin, heptaporphyrin (urine), ↑ isocoproporphyrin (faeces)
* *Hepatoerythropoietic porphyria*: uroporphyrinogen decarboxylase (*UROD* gene), aut. rec.: severe variant of PCT, same clinical picture as CEP
* *Congenital erythropoietic porphyria* (CEP, Günther disease): uroporphyrinogen-III synthase (*UROS* gene), aut. rec.; early onset (neonatal-childhood): dermatosis, tooth/bone changes, corneal scarring, haemolytic anaemia (fetal hydrops); typical discolouration of the urine (brown, red-fluorescent spots in the nappies)
* *Porphyria variegata* and *hereditary coproporphyria*: see above, acute porphyrias

Porphyrias with acute painful photosensitivity

Clinical: Sun-exposed skin (any age): burning, stinging, pruritus, oedema within minutes of sun exposure; chronic thickening/scarring; liver dysfunction

Diagn.: ↑ Protoporphyrins (erythrocytes, faeces)

Therapy: Photoprotection, β-carotene; liver complications: cholestyramine, bile acids

* *Erythropoietic protoporphyria*: ferrochelatase (*FECH* gene), pseudodominant inheritance (comp. heterozygous for severe mutation + common functional variant IVS3-48C, allele frequency up to 43% [Japan])
* *X-chromosomal protoporphyria*: erythroid-specific aminolaevulinate synthase activating mutations (*ALAS2* gene, Xp11.21; loss-of-function mutations cause X-linked sideroblastic anaemia); males and females equally affected

Lipoprotein metabolism

Biochemistry

Lipoproteins are the lipid transport vehicles of the blood. The core of these particles contains hydrophobic molecules incl. triglycerides and cholesterolesters whilst the surface is composed of hydrophilic, charged molecules such as phospholipids and cholesterol. **Apolipoproteins** which are attached to the particles are required for structural integrity (ApoB-100, ApoB-48, ApoA-I) and serve as ligands (ApoB-100, ApoE, ApoA-I) or cofactors (ApoC-II, ApoA-I, ApoA-IV) for specific enzymes. Lipoproteins are classified according to density into high-density lipoproteins (HDL), intermediate (IDL), low (LDL) and very low-density lipoproteins (VLDL) as well as chylomicrons.

Chylomicrons and VLDL represent the triglyceride-rich lipoproteins and are assembled in the Golgi apparatus of duodenal mucosa and hepatocytes, respectively. Chylomicrons serve as transport vehicles of triglycerides absorbed in the gut, are synthesised in large quantities after meals and enter the blood stream via lymphatic vessels. VLDL are synthesised by the liver and also supply the peripheral cells with triglycerides and (particularly after conversion into LDL) cholesterol. ApoC-II plays an important role in chylomicron and VLDL breakdown as the cofactor of *lipoproteinlipase* (a glycoprotein attached to the endothelium) which cleaves triglycerides into glycerol and fatty acids for further metabolism in the cell. The **remnants** of the chylomicrons are taken up by the liver (via the ApoE receptor) and metabolised. VLDL changes into **IDL** and after removal of further lipids finally turns into the cholesterol-rich LDL particles. If these are not required in the periphery they are taken up again by the liver via the LDL receptor.

LDL is found in several different subfractions (LDL1–LDL6); LDL 6 is described as a small, dense and highly atherogenic particle. LDL binds via ApoB-100 to the LDL receptor, is taken up by endocytosis and broken down in the lysosome, mainly by *acid lipase* (see *page 142*). Cholesterol ist released, inhibits the activity of *HMG-CoA synthase* (see *page 117*) and is stored via *acyl-CoA cholesterol acyltransferase* (ACAT) in the lipid droplets of the cell.

HDL is also found in different subfractions (HDL1–3). It is generated mainly by chylomicron metabolism and interaction with VLDL. Via ApoA-I (the major protein component) and ApoA-IV, HDL activates *lecithin:cholesterol acyltransferase* (LCAT), inducing enrichment with cholesterol esters. These may be exchanged for triglycerides of other lipoproteins via the exchange protein CETP. By this mechanism, most of the HDL cholesterol is metabolised via the LDL pathway. HDL is also taken up directly (mainly via ApoA-I) and broken down by the liver. HDL thereby serves as a transport vehicle for "reverse" cholesterol transport from peripheral cells back to the liver and has a vasoprotective effect.

Lipoprotein	Apolipoprotein (Apo)	Function
Chylomicrons	A-I, A-IV, C-I, C-II, C-III, E, B-48	Transport of exogenous triglycerides, fat soluble vitamins and drugs
VLDL	CI-III, E, B-100	Transport of endogenous triglycerides
IDL	CII, E, B-100	Product of VLDL triglyceride removal
LDL	B-100	Product of IDL triglyceride removal; cholesterol transport to extrahepatic tissue; regulation of cholesterol biosynthesis
HDL	A-I, A-II, A-IV, C-I, C-III, D, E	Mainly modification of other lipoproteins, cholesterol transport to the liver
Lipoprotein (a)	B-100, Apo (a)	Uncertain, possibly for vascular repair; risk factor for atherosclerosis

Hypercholesterolaemias

Familial hypercholesterolaemia (FH)

Clinical: *Heterozygous*: adult presentation – premature atherosclerosis, familial vascular disease (myocardial infarctions), xanthomas, xanthelasms, thickened tendons (e.g. Achilles tendon), arcus corneae

          Homozygous: severe atherosclerosis from early childhood; DD sitosterolaemia

Genetics: LDL receptor, *LDLR* gene, aut. semi-dom. inheritance, incidence: heterozygous ~1:500, homozygous

Diagn.:   ↑ Cholesterol (heterozygous ~300 mg/dl, homozygous >600 mg/dl), normal triglycerides, ↓ HDL; mutation analysis; *family history* (cholesterol >260 mg/dl + cardiovascular events in parents)

Procedure: *Total cholesterol > 200 mg/dl* (5.2 mmol/l), normal HDL (>35 mg/dl):
- LDL-cholesterol 110–130 mg/dl: check again within 2 yrs
- LDL-cholesterol >130 mg/dl (3.4 mmol/l): diet
- LDL-cholesterol >190 mg/dl (4.9 mmol/l) despite diet for 6–12 mths or >160 mg/dl (4.2 mmol/l) + positive family history: consider drug therapy
- LDL-cholesterol >250 mg/dl (6.5 mmol/l): transfer to metabolic centre

Therapy: *Diet*: (↓ cholesterol <200 mg/day, ↓ saturated fats <7–10% of energy intake); *drugs*: anion exchangers (cholestyramine), statins, etc.

          Homozygous patients: cholesterol removal via LDL apheresis (weekly to fortnightly); consider liver transplantation; gene therapy not yet successful

Follow up: 3–6-mthly during diet therapy

Familial ApoB-100 deficiency (FDB)

Clinical: Same as in LDLR deficiency; *homozygosity*: cholesterol level and cardiovascular risk as in heterozygotes (ApoB function partly replaced by ApoE)

Genetics: *APOB* gene, aut. semi-dom.; incidence: heterozygous ~1:300–700; missense mutations in the receptor binding region, e.g. p.R3500Q

Therapy: Same as in LDL receptor deficiency

Sitosterolaemia (= phytosterolaemia)

Clinical: Xanthomas, premature atherosclerosis (DD); occasionally haemolysis

Bioch.:   ↑ Intestinal absorption and ↓ biliary excretion of fish/plant sterols

Genetics: Aut. rec., *ABCG5* or *ABCG8* genes (twinned sterol half-transporters)

Diagn.:   n–↑↑ Cholesterol; ↑ phytosterols/sitosterols (serum, GC-MS)

Therapy: Effective diet therapy (↓ plant oils, etc.) and anion exchange resins

Other hypercholesterolaemias

- *Wolman disease*: lysosomal cholesterol-ester storage disease (see *page 142*)
- *Hyperlipoprotein(a) disease*
- *Hyperbetalipoproteinaemia*
- *Polygenic hypercholesterolaemia*
- *Secondary hypercholesterolaemia* in hypothyroidism, renal disease, Cushing syndrome, anorexia nervosa, acromegaly or increased STH secretion

Hypertriglyceridaemias

Familial chylomicronaemia (Frederickson HLP I or V)

Clinical: Abdominal complaints, failure to thrive, recurrent, sometimes fatal pancreatitis, hepatosplenomegaly, eruptive xanthomas; no increased risk of atherosclerosis; often asymptomatic

Enzyme: Lipoproteinlipase (*LPL* gene), rarely ApoC-II (*APOC2* gene)

Genetics: Aut. rec.; symptomatic carriers with additional risk factors

Bioch.:   Disorder of triglyceride breakdown from chylomicrons and VLDL

Diagn.:   ↑↑ Triglycerides (chylomicrons, VLDL) mostly > 500 mg/dl

DD: Drugs, alcohol, renal disease

Therapy: Very low (saturated) fat, avoid aggravating hormones (steroids, oestrogens); *acute*: lipid apheresis; in ApoC-II deficiency: supplement ApoC-II (in FFP)

Familial hypertriglyceridaemia

Clinical: Mostly asymptomatic; as "metabolic syndrome" associated with obesity, disturbed glucose tolerance, ↑ uric acid, hypertension

Genetics: Heterogenous; *APO5* gene, *LIPI* gene

Diagn.:   ↑ Triglycerides (VLDL, chylomicrons); sometimes peripheral insulin resistance

DD: Diabetes mellitus, Cushing syndrome, hypothyroidism, renal disease, etc.

Therapy: Symptomatic; diet, ↓ rapidly absorbed carbohydrates, consider drugs (fibrates, niacin, statins), fish oils, weight loss, regular exercise

Mixed hyperlipidaemias

Familial combined hyperlipidaemia (FCHL)

Clinical: Milder than LDL receptor deficiency

Bioch.:   Uncertain; overproduction of VLDL

Genetics: Heterogeneous (incl. *USF1* mutations); common: incidence up to 1:300

Diagn.:   ↑ Cholesterol and triglycerides; positive family history, alternating lipid profiles (triglycerides normal-pathological) within the family and over time

Therapy: Effective diet therapy (↓ rapidly absorbed carbohydrates), statins

Type III hyperlipidaemia (familial dysbetalipoproteinaemia)

Clinical: Xanthomas, xanthelasms, orange discolouration of hand creases; atherosclerosis; rare in children

Bioch.:   *APOE* gene variants → deficient IDL/remnant uptake in the liver

Genetics: Common: homozygosity for ApoE2 variant (aut. rec.); other mutations in the receptor binding domain (aut. dom.)

Incidence: 1:5,000

Diagn.:   ↑ Cholesterol and triglycerides, typical pattern in lipid electrophoresis

Therapy: Treat other risk factors (e.g. diabetes mellitus); diet; lipid lowering drugs

Other mixed hyperlipidaemias

• *Hepatic lipase deficiency*: similar to ApoE variants; *LIPC* gene, aut. rec.

Disorders of high density lipoprotein (HDL) metabolism

Hypoalphalipoproteinaemia ($\downarrow$ HDL, $\downarrow$ ApoA-I), often familial, is an important risk factor of premature atherosclerosis. The aetiology is freqeuntly unclear; secondary causes include hypertriglyceridaemia, liver failure, intestinal disorders, acute inflammation or certain drugs (e.g. steroids). Therapy is symptomatic through avoidance of other risk factors of atherosclerosis.

Apolipoprotein A-I deficiency

Clinical: Early atherosclerosis, xanthomas, corneal clouding; occasionally amyloidosis
Genetics: *APOA1* mutations, variable severity; some associated with familial amyloidosis
Diagn.: $\downarrow$ HDL, $\downarrow$ ApoA-I
Therapy: Avoid risk factors of atherosclerosis

Tangier disease, familial hypoalphalipoproteinaemia

Clinical: Polyneuropathy (weakness, paraesthesias, etc.); hyperplastic orange tonsils; hepatosplenomegaly, corneal clouding, coronary artery disease
Genetics: *ABCA1* gene; *Tangier*: aut. rec.; *familial hypoalphalipoproteinaemia*: heterozygous mutations (half normal HDL), often asymptomatic
Bioch.:   Generation of foam cells due to disturbed intracellular transport of cholesterol esters in macrophages
Diagn.: $\downarrow\downarrow$ HDL, $\downarrow$ ApoA-I, $\uparrow$ triglycerides, n–$\downarrow$ cholesterol

Lecithin:cholesterol acyltransferase deficiency

Clinical: Corneal clouding, nephropathy $\rightarrow$ renal failure, hypochromic anaemia
           Fish-eye disease: isolated corneal clouding
Genetics: *LCAT* gene, aut. rec.
Diagn.: $\downarrow$ HDL, $\downarrow$ ApoA-I, $\uparrow$ triglycerides, free/total cholesterol >0.7

Elevation of HDL

- *Familial hyperalphalipoproteinaemia*: cholesterol-ester transfer protein (CETP) deficiency $\rightarrow$ cholesterol-esters remain in HDL, $\uparrow$ HDL; clinically asymptomatic often increased life-span; *CETP* gene, semi-dominant
- *Secondary*: exercise, alcohol, drugs (e.g. oestrogens)

Disorders with decreased LDL cholesterol and triglycerides

Familial abetalipoproteinaemia

Clinical: Fat malabsorption (steatorrhoea, vomiting, failure to thrive); vit. E/A deficiencies (neuropathy, ataxia, cerebellar signs; retinopathy; myopathy)

Protein: Microsomal triglyceride transfer protein, *MTTP* gene, aut. rec.

Bioch.:   Deficient triglyceride transport into endoplasmic reticulum → deficient production of ApoB-containing lipoproteins; deficient transport capacity for fat-soluble vitamins and drugs; erythrocyte dysfunction

Diagn.:   ↓↓ Cholesterol and triglycerides; lack of ApoB; *blood smear*: acanthocytes (DD see *page 29*); normal cholesterol, triglycerides + ApoB in the parents

Therapy: Vit. E 100 mg/kg/day; vit. A, K, D (i.m.); very low fat diet

Familial hypobetalipoproteinaemia

Clinical: Like MTTP deficiency, but milder

Protein: Apolipoprotein B, *APOB* gene, aut. semi-dom.

Diagn.:   Like MTTP deficiency; parents ↓ cholesterol, triglycerides, ApoB

Chylomicron retention disease (Anderson)

Clinical: Fat malabsorption, failure to thrive, vitamin deficiency

Genetics: *SAR1B* gene, aut. rec., intracellular trafficking of chylomicrons in enterocytes

Diagn.:   ↓ Cholesterol, triglycerides, ApoA-I, ApoB; fat droplets in enterocytes

Lysosomal metabolism

Biochemistry
Lysosomes are required for the intracellular breakdown of various molecules and compounds of all sizes. For this purpose they contain a range of hydrolases in an acidic environment (pH 5). Some lysosomal enzymes are secreted and taken up by other cells through endocytosis and can therefore be measured in body fluids.

Genetic defects of lysosomal enzymes usually cause the accumulation of incompletely catabolised substrates within the organelle and progressive impairment of the function of affected cell systems (e.g. connective tissue, solid organs, cartilage, bone and, above all, nervous tissue). The cell and consequently the whole organ "swells", causing typical organomegaly and other morphological features. However, some conditions have specific other clinical symptoms not immediately recognised as "lysosomal".

Groups of disorders
- *Mucopolysaccharidoses* (*MPS*): deficient breakdown of glycosaminoglycans (GAGs)
- *Oligosaccharidoses*: deficient breakdown of carbohydrate side-chains from glycoproteins
- *Sphingolipidoses*: deficient breakdown of ceramide-containing membrane lipids
- *Neuronal ceroid lipofuscinoses*
- *Lysosomal export defects*
- *Other lysosomal disorders*

Typical findings in lysosomal storage diseases

Note: The clinical manifestations are generally variable.

	Coarse facial features	Dysostosis multiplex	Organomegaly	Intellectual disability	Spasticity	Peripheral neuropathy	Myoclonic seizures	Hydrops fetalis	Angiokeratoma	Corneal clouding	Cherry-red spot	Cardiac involvement	Macroglossia	Vacuolated lymphocytes	GAG (urine) elevated	Pathological oligosaccharides	Enzyme studies in: (discuss with laboratory)
Mucopolysaccharidoses																	
MPS type IH	++	++	+	++						++		+	++		+		L/F
MPS type IS	+	+	+							+		+	(+)		+		L/F
MPS type II	++	+	+	++								+	+		+		S/L/F
MPS type III	(+)	(+)	(+)	++	+					+					(+)		L/F
MPS type IV	+	a	+	(+)				+		(+)					(+)		L/F
MPS type VI	(+)	++	+							++		+	++		+		L/F
MPS type VII	+	+	+	+				+		(+)		+			+		S/L/F
MPS type IX	+	b				?											L/F
Oligosaccharidoses																	
Fucosidosis	+	(+)	(+)	++	+				+			(+)		+		+	S/L/F
α-Mannosidosis	++	+	+	++	(+)				(+)	++				+		+	S/L/F
β-Mannosidosis	+			+	+	+			(+)							+	S/L/F
Asp.glucosaminuria	+	(+)	(+)	+					(+)	(+)				(+)		+	L/F
Schindler				+	+		+									+	S/L/F
Sialidosis type I					+	+	++	+			++			+		+	F
Sialidosis type II	++	(+)	+	++			(+)	(+)	+		++			+		+	F

Legend

++ = prominent feature, + = often present, (+) = sometimes present; a = severe skeletal dysplasia but not classical DM, b = peri-articular swelling
- Angiokeratoma = red to dark blue lesions (< 1 mm, slightly hyperkeratotic, do not blanche on pressure) mostly on buttocks, genitalia, lower trunk, thighs)
- Cherry-red spot – in the macula region
- Cardiac involvement = cardiomyopathy, valve lesions, coronary artery disease
- Vacuolated lymphocytes = typical vacuoles or evidence of storage in lymphocytes

F = fibroblasts, L = leukocytes, S = serum, M = muscle

	Coarse facial features	Dysostosis multiplex	Organomegaly	Intellectual disability	Spasticity	Peripheral neuropathy	Myoclonic seizures	Hydrops fetalis	Angiokeratoma	Corneal clouding	Cherry-red spot	Cardiac involvement	Macroglossia	Vacuolated lymphocytes	GAG (urine) elevated	Pathological oligosaccharides	Enzyme studies in: (discuss with laboratory)
Sphingolipidoses																	
GM₁ gangliosidosis	++	+	+	++	(+)			+	+	+	++	(+)	+			+	L/F
GM₂ gangliosidosis			(+)	++	+		+				++					(+)	S/L/F
Galactosialidosis	++	++	++	++	+		(+)	+	(+)	+	+	+		+		–/+	F
MLD				++	+	++					(+)						L/F
Niemann-Pick A, B			++	+				(+)	+	(+)	(+)			+			L/F
Gaucher type I			+													(+)	L/F
Gaucher type II			+	++	+		+	+								(+)	L/F
Gaucher type III			+	+	(+)		(+)	(+)				(+)				(+)	L/F
Fabry									+			+					S/L/F
Krabbe				++	+	++					(+)						L/F
Farber			+	+			+			(+)	(+)						F
Multiple sulphatase deficiency	++	++	++	++	++		+			+	(+)	+	+		+		L/F
Mucolipidoses																	
Mucolipidosis II	++	++	+	++						+		++	+	+			S/F
Mucolipidosis III	(+)	(+)	(+)	(+)								++		+			S/F
Mucolipidosis IV				+	+							+	+	+			F
Lipid storage diseases																	
Niemann-Pick C + D			(+)	+	+	+					(+)			+			F
Wolman			+					+			(+)	(+)		+			L
Lysosomal transport defects																	
Cystinosis			(+)							+							L
Sialic acid storage	(+)	(+)	(+)	+		+	(+)							+		–	–
Neuronal ceroid lipofuscinoses (incl. Batten disease)																	
Infantile				+	+		+							(+)			L/F
Late infantile				+	+		+							(+)			L/F
Juvenile				+			(+)							+			
Adult				+	(+)		(+)							(+)			
Glycogen storage disease type II																	
Pompe (*page 84*)			+									++	+	+		(+)	L/F/M

Diagnosis
There is substantial clinical overlap between different disorders, and the age of manifestation may be variable.

Symptoms and signs
- Chronic progression of symptoms without acute metabolic crises
- In the *neonatal period* often (but not always) unremarkable; sometimes hydrops fetalis, dysmorphic facies, cardiomegaly
- Initially often muscular hypotonia, motor delay and later intellectual disability
- Progressive organomegaly (liver, spleen, heart)
- Coarse facial features, skeletal changes, skin changes
- Ataxia, hyperexcitability, spasticity in neurological storage disorders
- Cherry-red spot in the macula region in some disorders

Investigations
- Examine skeleton (X-ray lateral skull, lateral lumbar spine, hand, pelvis; dysostosis multiplex?)
- Examine parenchymatous organs (ultrasound) and heart (ECG, echo)
- Check eyes (retina, macula, lens, cornea), hearing; consider cranial MRI scan
- Check for vacuoles in leukocytes (reliably found only in *immediate* blood smear; do not use blood from an EDTA tube!), bone marrow cells or biopsies
- Analyse glycosaminoglycans and oligosaccharides in the urine
- If indicated, measure enzyme activities in leukocytes or fibroblasts
- Check chitotriosidase activity (serum, dried blood spot)
- High sensitivity in EM of skin fibroblasts (distended lysosomes)

Chitotriosidase is a chitinolytic enzyme and marker of monocyte/macrophage activation. It is highly elevated in some lysosomal storage disorders incl. Gaucher, Niemann-Pick A/B and C diseases and can be useful for screening and/or monitoring of treatment.

Note: False negative results in patients homozygous for a common null allele of the *CHIT1* gene (6% of Caucasians). Chitotriosidase activity is also increased in a large number of non-metabolic conditions incl. atherosclerosis, sarcoidosis, beta-thalassaemia or malaria.

Curative therapy
- *Haematopoietic stem cell transplantation* (HSCT) has proven benefit in presymptomatic patients in some disorders (e.g. MPS I, late-onset Krabbe disease, metachromatic leukodystrophy) but not in others (MPS III, MPS IV).
- *Enzyme replacement therapy* (ERT) is licensed and available for Gaucher, Fabry, and Pompe disease as well as MPS I, II and VI. Clinical trials are in progress for MPS IV A, and trials with intrathecal ERT are in progress for the neuronopathic form of MPS II and IIIA (peripheral administration is not effective for cerebral disease manifestations as the enzyme does not cross the blood-brain barrier).

Mucopolysaccharidoses (MPS)

Mucopolysaccharidoses are disorders in the breakdown of glycosaminoglycans (GAG). These are long chains of sulphated or acetylated (amino) sugars attached to a protein skeleton. They constitute the viscous extracellular matrix.

Clinical: Affected children usually appear normal at birth but (in most MPS) subsequently develop progressive *connective tissue changes* (facial dysmorphism, skin changes) *skeletal deformities* (growth restriction, bone dysplasia, contractures), as well as *hepatomegaly* and often hernias. Depending on the MPS type there may be *progressive psychomotor retardation* with loss of acquired skills, corneal clouding, and deafness. Obstructive and restrictive *airway disease* (incl. recurrent upper and lower respiratory tract infections) and *cardiac disease* (valvular dysfunction, cardiomyopathy, pulmonary hypertension) are common. Type II MPS (Hunter) is an X-chromosomal disease.

Diagnosis: Primarily by the analysis of glycosaminoglycans (GAG, previously called mucopolysaccharides) in the urine (best and reliable by GAG electrophoresis; *caution*: screening tests may give false negative results, particularly in types III, IV and IX); confirmation by enzyme analysis (leukocytes, fibroblasts) and molecular studies.

Treatment: Enzyme replacement therapy is effective for non-cerebral manifestations in MPS I, II, VI (and possibly IV). Haematopoietic stem cell transplant (HSCT) has proven benefit in presymptomatic patients with severe MPS I and MPS VI, and anecdotal benefit in a few patients with MPS II. Otherwise, treatment is largely symptomatic.

Pathological glycosaminoglycans in different MPS and multiple sulphatase deficiency

	Normal	Mucopolysaccharidosis							Mult. sulph. def.	Typical clinical findings, affected organ systems
		I	II	III	IV	VI	VII	IX		
Dermatan sulphate		++	++			++	n–+		++	Skeleton + internal organs
Heparan sulphate		+	+	+			n–+		++	Intellectual disability
Keratan sulphate					+					Skeleton
Chondroitin sulphate	+				(+)		+	++	++	

MPS type I (Hurler, Scheie)

Enzyme: α-L-Iduronidase (*IDUA* gene)

Hurler: Severe form (MPS1H), onset in first year with recurrent upper respiratory tract infections → slowing of growth and psychomotor development, progressive hepatosplenomegaly, dysmorphism, cardiac disease, corneal clouding (>age 1), hydrocephalus; fatal within 5–10 yrs

Scheie: Milder form (MPS1S), onset in adolescence and adulthood: normal intelligence, mostly normal height; mild skeletal deformities, degenerative joint disease, corneal clouding, cardiac valve lesion

Intermediate form: Hurler-Scheie disease (MPS1H/S), onset in school age

Therapy: Enzyme replacement for non-cerebral symptoms (Laronidase [Aldurazyme®]); BMT/HSCT should be considered in young patients (below age 2 yrs)

MPS type II (Hunter)

Enzyme: Iduronate-2-sulphatase (X-chromosomal, *IDS* gene)
Clinical: Joint contractures, obstructive and restrictive airway disease, cardiac disease, skeletal deformities, progressive cognitive decline; fatal within 10–20 yrs (respiratory/cardiac failure). No corneal clouding. Around $^1/_3$ of patients have an attenuated (adult) form with normal intelligence and milder somatic features (progressive retinal dysfunction, spastic paresis, severe hip disease, cardiac complications).
           Female carriers are usually asymptomatic.
Therapy: Enzyme replacement for non-cerebral symptoms (Idursulfase [Elaprase®])

MPS type III (Sanfilippo)

Enzyme: 4 Enzymes of heparan sulphate metabolism (genes: type A = *SGSH*, type B = *NAGLU*, type C = *HGSNAT*, type D = *GNS*), C + D are less common
Clinical: Encephalopathy with minor organ involvement: developmental/language delay in infancy → behavioural disturbances, hyperactivity, sleep disorders, intellectual disability, seizures → neurodegeneration, tetraspasticity by age 10–30. Normal height, mild dysostosis. Attenuated forms with later onset.

MPS type IV (Morquio)

Enzyme: 2 Enzymes of keratan sulphate metabolism (genes: type A = *GALNS*, frequent; type B = *GLB1*, also mutated in GM_1-gangliosidosis)
Clinical: Normal intelligence, small stature, severe skeletal deformities, atlanto-axial instability

Other mucopolysaccharidoses

Type VI: *Maroteaux-Lamy disease*: deficient N-acetylgalactosamine-4-sulphatase (arylsulphatase B, *ARSB* gene); normal intelligence, skeletal deformities similar to Hurler disease, recognised from age 2 onwards; often macrocephaly at birth; early diagnosis important for ERT (galsulfase [Naglazyme®])
Type VII: *Sly disease*: deficient β-glucuronidase (*GUSB* gene), usually like Hurler disease with dysostosis multiplex, hepatosplenomegaly; broad spectrum ranging from hydrops fetalis to almost normal
Type IX: *Natowicz disease*: deficient hyaluronidase (*HYAL1* gene); one reported patient with short stature and multiple painful peri-articular soft-tissue masses; ↑ hyaluronidase in blood (GAGs may be normal)

Oligosaccharidoses

Oligosaccharidoses are disorders in the breakdown of complex carbohydrate side-chains of gly-cosylated proteins (glycoproteins; for their biosynthesis see CDG *page 146*).

Clinical: Oligosaccharidoses resemble MPS but are less common. *Skeletal deformities* and *coarse facies* may range from severe to mild. There is usually *intellectual disability*, often with behav-ioural difficulties, progressive neurological symptoms and seizures. Hepatomegaly, deafness and corneal clouding may be absent; some disorders (especially sialidosis) show a *cherry-red macula spot*. Early manifestation is more frequent than in the MPS: Some disorders present at birth or in the first year (hydrops fetalis, cardiomegaly) and are often fatal within a few years (or earlier). Severity may vary greatly depending on the individual mutation.

Diagnosis: Primarily by increased urinary excretion of oligosaccharides (also observed in GM_1 gangliosidosis, GM_2 gangliosidosis [Tay-Sachs, Sandhoff] and galactosialidosis); GAGs are nor-mal, urinary neuraminic acid is elevated in sialidosis. Some conditions show vacuolated lym-phocytes. Confirmation by enzyme analysis (leukocytes, fibroblasts; see table) and molecular stud-ies.

Treatment: Symptomatic; haematopoietic stem cell transplant in α-mannosidosis.

α-Mannosidosis
Enzyme: α-Mannosidase; *MAN2B1* gene
Clinical: *Severe form* (*type I*): Hurler-like disease, progressive intellectual disability; deafness, cataract, corneal clouding, hydrocephalus, progressive ataxia, dysostosis multiplex, hernias, hepatomegaly; immune deficiency (frequent bacterial infections); rapidly pro-gressive, fatal within first decade
Attenuated form (*type II*) with manifestation in childhood or adolescence

Sialidosis
This disease is traditionally classified as mucolipidosis type I but is essentially an oligo-saccharidosis. In combination with β-galactosidase deficiency: galactosialidosis (*page 142*; Cathepsin A).
Enzyme: Acid sialidase (α-neuraminidase; *NEU1* gene)
Type I: Cherry-red spot-myoclonus syndrome: ↓ vision, gait abnormalities, seizures; onset in adolescence or early adulthood
Type II: Progressive psychomotor retardation, facial dysmorphism, kyphosis in early child-hood, deafness, progressive ataxia, myoclonus
Neonatal: Congenital non-immune hydrops

Other Oligosaccharidoses
- *β-Mannosidosis*: deficient β-mannosidase (*MANBA* gene), intellectual disability, behavioural difficulties, peripheral neuropathy, angiokeratomas (adults)
- *Fucosidosis*: deficient α-Fucosidase (*FUCA1* gene); neurodegeneration, epilepsy, mild to se-vere hepatosplenomegaly, mild dysostosis; widespread angiokeratomas
- *Schindler disease*: deficient α-N-Acetylgalactosaminidase = α-galactosidase B (*NAGA* gene); Neurodegeneration, myoclonic epilepsy
- *Aspartylglucosaminuria*: deficient aspartylglucosaminase (*AGA* gene); neurodegeneration, con-nective tissue changes, mild hepatosplenomegaly

Sphingolipidoses

Sphingolipids are major components of cellular membranes. They consist of ceramide (sphingosine + long-chain fatty acid) which serves as a hydrophobic anchor for (mostly polar) residues e.g. on the outside of the cell. Some sphingolipids are thought to have protective functions while others are required e.g. for cell recognition and signalling. Sphingolipids are found throughout the body but are of special importance in the nervous tissue, and most sphingolipidoses present with primary disturbances in the central or peripheral nervous system. In addition, sphingolipids frequently accumulate in the reticuloendothelial system or other cells.

- *Glycosphingolipids* = ceramide + carbohydrate side chain (one or more sugars)
  - *Gangliosides* = ceramide + 3–7 carbohydrates, one of which is sialic acid (N-acetylneuraminic acid); common e.g. in the grey matter of the brain
  - *Cerbrosides* = ceramide + single sugar (galactocerebrosides mainly in neural tissue, glucocerebrosides in various tissues)
  - *Sulphatides* = sulphated cerebrosides, essential components of myelin sheaths
- *Sphingomyelin* = ceramide + phosphocholine (or phosphoethanolamine)

Clinical features include *progressive psychomotor retardation, neurological problems*, specifically *epilepsy* as well as ataxia and/or spasticity. *Hepatosplenomegaly* is not uncommon, dysmorphism or skeletal deformities are rare (except in GM$_1$ gangliosidosis). Some disorders show a cherry-red macula spot, foam cells in the bone marrow or vacuolated lymphocytes. Neurological and neuroradiological findings are not always specific; clinically distinct *lysosomal leukodystrophies* are the metachromatic leukodystrophy and Krabbe disease.

Diagnosis: Enzyme analyses are possible in fibroblasts and often leukocytes (or serum); see table. Some conditions show elevated oligosaccharides in the urine.

GM$_1$ gangliosidosis

Acid β-galactosidase removes galactose from GM$_1$ gangliosides as well as some oligosaccharides and keratan sulphate. Mutations in its gene *GLB1* may cause both GM$_1$ gangliosidosis and Morquio disease type B (see *page 134*). The protein functions in a multi-enzyme complex and is also deficient in galactosialidosis (*page 142*; Cathepsin A).

Enzyme: β-Galactosidase (*GLB1* gene)

Type I: Neonatal hypotonia, sometimes oedema (occasionally fetal hydrops), facial dysmorphism; arrest of neurological development → decerebration; hepatosplenomegaly, scoliosis, dysostosis multiplex, blindness (nystagmus), 50% cherry-red spot (rarely before age 6 mths), death often before age 2

Type II: Late infantile/juvenile presentation with ataxia → quadriparesis; no dysmorphism, mild bone changes, no hepatosplenomegaly

Type III: Chronic/adult presentation with dystonia, cerebellar dysarthria, ataxia; no bone changes; cognition normal or moderately impaired

Diagn.: Vacuolated lymphocytes (not always); oligosaccharides/GAG (urine)

GM$_2$ gangliosidosis (Tay-Sachs disease, Sandhoff disease)

Breakdown of GM$_2$ gangliosides requires GM$_2$ activator protein and β-hexosaminidase A (αβ-heterodimer). Hexosaminidase B (ββ-homodimer) hydrolyses other substrates with terminal hexosamines (e.g. in glycoproteins).

- *Tay Sachs* (B variant): deficient β-hexosaminidase A (α-subunit, *HEXA* gene)
- *Sandhoff* (0 variant); deficient β-hexosaminidase A + B (β-subunit, *HEXB* gene)
- *GM$_2$ activator protein deficiency* ("variant AB", *GM2A* gene); rare

Clinical: *Infantile form*: onset at age 4–6 mths: hypotonia, startle reaction, cherry-red spot →
             blindness, spastic tetraparesis, decerebration; macrocephaly from 18 mths onwards;
             hepatosplenomegaly may be found in Sandhoff disease
             Late infantile/juvenile form: ataxia, incoordination, dysarthria, myoclonus
             Chronic/adult forms: movement disorder, neurological/psychiatric symptoms

Diagn.:   Patients with Sandhoff disease may have vacuolated lymphocytes or elevated urinary
             oligosaccharides. Hexosaminidase A and B activities are both normal in GM$_2$ activator protein deficiency.

Metachromatic leukodystrophy (MLD)

Enzyme: Sulphatidase = arylsulphatase A (*ARSA* gene)

Clinical: *Lysosomal leukodystrophy* with central and peripheral demyelination: onset age 1–2
             with spasticity (equinus position of feet), neuropathy, loss of skills (e.g. walking) →
             optic atrophy, tetraspasticity, decerebration; fatal age 3–6
             Juvenile form with onset age 6–8; *adult form*

Diagn.:   Often ↑ CSF protein; ↓ nerve conduction velocity; ↑ sulphatides (urine); *enzyme studies*: beware of pseudo-deficiency (↓↓ amount of enzyme protein in 1–2% of Europeans,
             clinically irrelevant)

Therapy: HSCT in pre-symptomatic or early symptomatic juvenile onset patients

Variants: • *Saposin B deficiency*: see *page 139*; ↑ sulphatides, glycolipids as in Fabry
             • *Multiple sulphatase deficiency*: MLD + Hurler-like disease + ichthyosis; deficient
               formylglycine generating enzyme (SUMF1 gene)

Krabbe disease (globoid cell leukodystrophy)

Enzyme: Galactosylceramidase (β-Galactocerebrosidase; *GALC* gene)

Clinical: *Lysosomal leukodystrophy* with central and peripheral demyelination: onset age 3–6
             mths with irritability, feeding problems, startle reaction, neuropathy, fever, spasticity,
             → blindness, deafness, decerebration; fatal before age 2
             Juvenile form (10%): progressive ataxia, spastic paraparesis, visual failure

Diagn.:   ↑ CSF protein concentration (not in late forms); ↓ nerve conduction velocity

Therapy: HSCT possibly not completely effective even in pre-symptomatic infants identified by
             newborn screening

Variants: *Saposin A deficiency* (see *page 139*)

Niemann-Pick disease types A and B

Enzyme: Sphingomyelinase (*SMPD1* gene)
Type A: Neonatal onset: feeding problems, hypotonia, failure to thrive, lymphadenopathy, hepatosplenomegaly → neurological deterioration, deafness, blindness; cherry-red spot (50%); fatal within 1.5–3 yrs
Type B: (Hepato)splenomegaly usually detected in late infancy or childhood, interstitial lung disease, growth restriction; normal intelligence and life span
Diagn.:   Atherogenic lipid profiles, mild liver dysfunction, low platelet count; foam cells "Niemann-Pick cells" in bone marrow

Niemann-Pick disease type C

Bioch.:   Disorder of cellular cholesterol trafficking → cholesterol storage; secondary storage of sphingomyelin and glycosphingolipids
           NPC1 gene: late endosomal membrane protein (90% of cases)
           NPC2 gene: lysosomal cholesterol-binding protein
Clinical: *Late infantile* (*juvenile*) presentation age 3–5(–15) yrs with progressive ataxia, language delay, behavioural problems, hepatosplenomegaly → intellectual decline, vertical supranuclear (upward) gaze palsy, cherry-red spot (50%), epilepsy, spasticity; cataplexy, dysphagia, dystonia; fatal by age 7–12(–adult)
Variants: *Foetal hydrops*
           Neonatal liver disease (30%) usually improves, may be fatal in infancy
           Adult onset: ataxia, dystonia, psychiatric symptoms, hepatomegaly, dementia
Diagn.:   Positive Filipin stain (cholesterol) in fibroblasts "Niemann-Pick cells" (sea blue histiocytes) in bone marrow; cholesterol esterification studies (fibroblasts)
Therapy: Substrate inhibition therapy (Miglustat [Zavesca®]) may decrease disease progression in some patients (approved in Europe for NPC treatment); HSCT may be effective in early diagnosed patients with NPC2 mutations

Gaucher disease

Enzyme: β-Glucosidase (Glucocerebrosidase; *GBA* gene)
Type I: *Non-neuronopathic form*, manifestation in infancy to adulthood with visceral, haematological and skeletal symptoms: severe (hepato)splenomegaly → anaemia, thrombocytopenia, bleeding tendency, acute abdominal pain (splenic infarctions); acute bone crises (painful medullary infarctions, osteonecrosis), osteopenia, fractures; growth restriction; lung fibrosis; normal intelligence, no CNS involvement
Type II: *Acute neuronopathic form*, rapidly progressive in infancy: brainstem dysfunction (ophthalmoplegia, dysphagia), spasticity, hepatosplenomegaly → CNS degeneration, cachexia, fatal within 1–2 yrs
Type III: *Chronic neuronopathic form*: between type I and II
Diagn.:   ↑ AP (acid phosphatase); "Gaucher cells" in bone marrow; chitotriosidase (in serum/plasma also for treatment monitoring)
Therapy: Enzyme replacement (primarily in visceral disease; imiglucerase [Cerezyme®], velaglucerase [VPRIV™]); substrate reduction (Miglustat [Zavesca®]); splenectomy in case of mechanical problems
Variants: *Saposin C deficiency*: see *page 139*; type III disease, rare

Fabry disease

Enzyme: Ceramide trihexosidase = α-galactosidase A
Genetics: X-chromosomal (*GLA* gene)
Clinical: Manifestation in the 1st decade: recurrent acute pain/paraesthesias in limbs, provoked
          by stress/temperature changes, lasting hours-days; recurrent fever, hypohidrosis; an-
          giokeratomas (80%), angiectasis, normal intelligence
          Adult complications: cardiomyopathy, renal failure; stroke, hearing loss
          Females: 70% are symptomatic; more variable, later onset
Diagn.:   Enzyme studies unreliable in females; ↑ urinary Gb3, Gb2 (glycolipids)
Therapy: Enzyme replacement (agalsidase alfa/beta [Replagal®, Fabrazyme®])

Farber disease (lipogranulomatosis, ceramidosis)

Enzyme: Ceramidase (*ASAH* gene)
Clinical: Painful contractures/joint deformities, hoarseness, skin nodules, neurodegeneration;
          infantile form fatal in 1–4 yrs; also juvenile forms
Therapy; HSCT

Saposin-related disorders

Hydrolysis of several sphingolipids requires the presence of four small glycoproteins called sa-
posins A–D. They are generated by cleavage of the four homologous domains of a single precur-
sor, prosaposin (*PSAP* gene). Deficiencies cause variant sphingolipidoses:
• Saposin A: activates galactosylceramidase (→ variant Krabbe disease)
• Saposin B: activates arylsulfatase A and others (→ variant MLD)
• Saposin C: activates β-glucosidase (→ variant Gaucher disease)
Combined deficiency: neonatal manifestation with severe neurological symptoms, hepatospleno-
megaly, rapidly fatal

Neuronal ceroid lipofuscinoses (NCL, CLN)

Neuronal ceroid lipofuscinoses are among the most common neurometabolic disorders.

Clinical:	• Seizures (often myoclonic); EEG changes may be specific
	• Progressive deterioration of cognition (loss of skills, dementia)
	• Motor dysfunction (involuntary movement, ataxia, spasticity)
	• Progressive loss of vision (retinopathy, optic atrophy), nystagmus
	• Deceleration of head growth, microcephaly
Bioch.:	Storage of autofluorescent lipid pigments (= ceroid) containing saposins A and C (CLN1, 10) or subunit C of the mitochondrial ATP synthase (other forms)
Diagn.:	(*Electron*)*microscopy* (skin biopsy, lymphocytes): distinct storage patterns; vacuolated lymphocytes (CLN3); enzyme studies (CLN1, 2, 10)
Therapy:	Symptomatic

Type	Protein	Gene	Typical presentation
CLN1	Palmitoyl protein thioesterase I	PPT1	Infantile (common in Finland)
CLN2	Tripeptidyl peptidase I	TPP1	Late infantile
CLN3	Lysosomal membrane protein	CLN3	Juvenile
CLN4	?	?	
CLN5	Soluble lysosomal protein	CLN5	
CLN6	Endoplasmic reticulum protein	CLN6	
CLN7	Lysosomal membrane protein	MFSD8	
CLN8	Endoplasmic reticulum protein	CLN8	
CLN9	?	?	
CLN10	Cathepsin D	CTSD	Any age incl. congenital

Congenital NCL
Manifestation at birth with microcephaly and seizures; rare; *CTSD* gene

Infantile NCL (Santavuori-Haltia disease)
Manifestation age 6–24 mths with developmental delay/regression, behavioural changes, poor co-ordination, poor speech, myoclonic jerks, deceleration of head growth, specific EEG changes →
retinal blindness, seizures; rapidly progressive, fatal within first decade.
• Genes: *PPT1*; common mutation in Finland

Late infantile NCL (Jansky-Bielschowsky disease)
Manifestation age 2–4(–7) yrs with epilepsy, developmental delay/regression, ataxia, extrapyra-midal/pyramidal signs, loss of vision (noticed at age 4–6); variable course with death in late child-hood or later (adulthood).
• Genes: *TPP1*; less frequently *CLN5* (Finland), *CLN6*, *MFSD8*, *CLN8*, *PPT1*, *CTSD*
• *Northern Epilepsy*: tonic-clonic/complex-partial seizures, motor dysfunction, slow cognitive decline throughout adulthood; *CLN8* mutation p.Arg24Gly (Finland)

Juvenile form (Batten disease, Vogt-Spielmeyer disease)
Manifestation age 4–10 yrs, often rapid loss of vision → blindness; epilepsy, regression, behavioural disturbances, hallucinations, disturbed sleep patterns, Parkinson disease-like rigor; life expectancy late adolescence-adulthood
• Genes: *CLN3*; less frequently *PPT1, TPP1, CLN9*

Adult NCL (Kufs disease)
Manifestation in adulthood: progressive myoclonic epilepsy, behavioural changes, dementia, ataxia, late-occurring pyramidal/extrapyramidal signs; fatal within 10 yrs
• Aut. rec. genes: *CTSD, PPT1, CLN3, CLN5, CLN4*
• Aut. dom. variant: rare, unknown gene

Lysosomal export defects

This group of disorders is characterised by failure to transport certain compounds released within the lysosomes across the lysosomal membrane and also includes the cblF defect in cobalamin metabolism (deficient lysosomal cobalamin release; see *page 156*).

Cystinosis
Bioch: Cystinosin deficiency (lysosomal cystin transporter *CTNS* gene)
Clinical: *Infantile*: nephropathy (tubulopathy, electrolyte disturbances) → renal failure; endocrine disturbances, small stature; sometimes hepatosplenomegaly, myopathy; corneal crystals (photophobia); later progressive central nervous symptoms (adulthood)
            Juvenile: nephropathy
            Adult: benign; corneal crystals
Diagn.:   Cystine content of leukocytes
Therapy: Symptomatic (Fanconi syndrome), cysteamine (10–)50 mg/kg/day, cysteamine eye drops
Progn.:   Good response to early treatment but late complications frequent

Sialic acid storage disease (Salla disease)
Bioch: Sialin deficiency (sialic [N-acetylneuraminic] acid transport, *SLC17A5* gene)
Clinical: Hypotonia, ataxia, mental and growth retardation, spasticity, epilepsy
            Infantile sialic acid storage disease, ISSD: fatal in infancy
            Salla disease: later onset, relatively long life-span, prevalent in Finland
Diagn.:   Free sialic acid (N-acetylneuraminic acid) in urine
DD: *Sialuria*: ↑ sialic acid biosynthesis due to deficient feedback inhibition (UDP-GlcNAc 2-epimerase, *GNE* gene); intellectual disability, mild dysmorphism, hepatosplenomegaly, occasionally seizures, mild dysostosis, normal growth; other *GNE* mutations cause aut. rec. inclusion body (Nonaka) myopathy

Other lysosomal disorders

Mucolipidoses (ML)
Mucolipidoses combine clinical features of MPS and sphingolipidoses. Mucolipidosis type I (ML-I) has been used as a term for sialidosis (see above).

I-cell disease (ML-II) and Pseudo-Hurler dystrophy (ML-III))
Enzyme: N-acetylglucosamine-1-phosphotransferase; $\alpha\alpha\beta\beta\gamma\gamma$-hexamer; genes: *GNPTA*: α/β-subunits (ML-II, ML-III); *GNPTG*: γ-subunit (ML-III)
Bioch.:   Deficiency of multiple lysosomal enzymes due to deficient post-translational modification in the Golgi apparatus for transport into lysosomes
Clinical: ML-II: Hurler-like, but earlier (neonatal) onset, fatal in early childhood
           ML-III: Hurler-like, onset age 2–4
Diagn.:   n–↑ GAGs (urine); activity of lysosomal enzymes: serum, plasma (fibroblasts)

Mucolipidosis type IV
Enzyme: Mucolipidin 1 (*MCOLN1* gene; Ca^{2+} channel, ? involved in endocytosis)
Clinical: Presentation in infancy with psychomotor delay, progressive loss of vision (corneal clouding + retinal degeneration), achlorhydria (↑ gastrin)
Diagn.:   ↑ Gastrin is useful screening test; ubiquitous vacuolar and avacuolar storage of gangliosides and lipopigment-like bodies

Wolman disease
Enzyme: Acid lipase (*LIPA* gene), cleaves cholesterol esters e.g. from LDL; *page 124*
Bioch.:   Lysosomal storage of cholesteryl esters and triglycerides
Clinical: Neonatal presentation with diarrhoea, vomiting, steatorrhoea, failure to thrive, hepatosplenomegaly, later anaemia, psychomotor retardation; typical adrenal enlargement and calcifications; usually fatal in infancy
Var.:   *Cholesteryl ester storage disease*: adults with hepatomegaly, fatty liver, lymphoadenopathy, hyperlipidaemia, increased transaminases, low HDL
Diagn.:   ↑ Cholesterol (serum); enzyme studies: leukocytes
Therapy: HMG-CoA reductase inhibitor for the treatment of atherosclerosis

Danon disease
Genetics: X-chromosomal
Bioch.:   Lysosome-associated membrane protein 2 (*LAMP2* gene)
Clinical: *Males*: like Pompe disease, childhood onset: cardiomyopathy, dysrhythmias (WPW syndrome), myopathy, intellectual disability, hepatopathy; often fatal in early adulthood
           Females: symptomatic but later onset, normal intelligence

Cathepsin-related disorders
Cathepsins are a large group of (mostly) lysosomal proteases with different functions.
- *Cathepsin A* (*PPGB* gene): multicatalytic with a variety of functions incl. processing of enzyme precursors and protection of β-galactosidase and sialidase → *galactosialidosis*: combined clinical and laboratory features of sialidosis and GM_1 gangliosidosis
- *Cathepsin C* (*CTSC* gene): removes N-terminal dipeptides from proteins and peptides → *Papillon-Lefevre syndrome*: keratosis palmoplantaris, severe periodontitis
- *Cathepsin K* (*CTSK* gene): proteinase involved in bone resorption → *pycnodysostosis*: facial dysmorphism, bone fragility

Peroxisomal metabolism

Biochemistry

Important peroxisomal functions include: β-oxidation of very long-chain fatty acids, pristanic acid, and intermediates of bile acid synthesis; α-oxidation of 3-methyl fatty acids (e.g. phytanic acid); biosynthesis of etherlipids (special phospholipids that occur mainly in the CNS, heart and skeletal muscle, e.g. plasmalogens); and glyoxylate detoxification. Many oxygen-dependent reactions take place in the peroxisomes to protect the cell against oxygen radicals; the produced H_2O_2 is metabolised by a catalase. Various *peroxins* encoded by *PEX* genes are required for peroxisome biogenesis and transmembrane transport. Peroxisomal proteins contain one of at least two different targeting signals (PTS1 and 2) for peroxisomal import.

Clinical features

- *Neurological abnormalities* – severe hypotonia, encephalopathy, seizures, deafness, retinopathy, cataract, blindness, etc.
- *Skeletal abnormalities*, in particular short proximal limbs; X-ray: calcific stippling
- *Dysmorphic features* (severe forms) – high forehead, very large fontanels, shallow supraorbital ridges, epicanthic folds, micrognathia, minor ear anomalies
- *Hepatointestinal dysfunction* – neonatal hepatitis, hepatomegaly, cholestasis, cirrhosis, etc.

Investigations

- Routine: n–↓ cholesterol, n–↑ bilirubin, abnormal liver function tests
- *Very long-chain fatty acids* (VLCFA, serum): ↑ C_{26}, etc. – indicates deficient peroxisomal β-oxidation, found in the majority of peroxisomal disorders
- *Plasmalogens* (erythrocytes): reduced in disorders affecting etherlipid biosynthesis
- *Phytanic acid* (serum): elevation indicates deficient α-oxidation, as in Refsum disease (dietary origin [meat], therefore always low = "normal" in neonates)
- *Pristanic acid* (serum, non-neonates): reduced in α-oxidation disorders, increased in β-oxidation disorders, isolated increase in α-methyl-acyl-CoA racemase deficiency
- *Bile acid intermediates* (serum, urine): increased intermediary products (see *page 120*)
- Enzyme studies, mutation analyses

	VLCFA	Plasma-logens	Phytanic acid	Pristanic acid	Bile acids
Disorders of peroxisomal biogenesis and beta-oxidation	↑	↓ or n	↑ or n	↑–n	↑–n
Rhizomelic chondrodysplasia punctata	n	↓	n–↑	↓–n	n
X-linked adrenoleukodystrophy	↑	n	n	n	n
Refsum disease	n	n	↑	↓	n
α-Methyl-acyl-CoA racemase deficiency	n	n	(↑)	↑	↑

Disorders of peroxisome biogenesis (Zellweger spectrum disorders)

Defective peroxisome assembly resulting in the deficiency of various enzymes, caused by mutations in one of the multiple *PEX* genes (>60% *PEX1*, otherwise *PEX2, 3, 5, 6, 10, 12, 13, 14, 16, 19, 26*). Depending on clinical presentation, variants are described as:

- *Zellweger syndrome*: neonatal presentation with severe hypotonia, areactivity, seizures, liver dysfunction (severe jaundice, cholestasis, ↑ conjugated bilirubin), dysmorphic and skeletal abnormalities, sensorineural deafness, retinopathy, cataracts, failure to thrive; MRI: pachypolymicrogyria; fatal within a few mths
- *Neonatal adrenoleukodystrophy*: somewhat less severe, neonatal or early infantile onset, hypotonia, seizures, hepatopathy (jaundice, hepatomegaly, portal hypertension), mild dysmorphic features, failure to thrive, gastrointestinal symptoms (vomiting, diarrhoea), osteoporosis, retinopathy → blindness, sensorineural deafness, progressive white matter disease, slower progression, fatal usually in late infancy
- *Infantile Refsum disease*: least severe variant, onset in (early) childhood, failure to thrive, liver disease, osteoporosis, variable cognitive/motor deficiencies, variable neurological symptoms/retinopathy/deafness, MRI may be unremarkable

Diagn.:   Evidence of multiple peroxisomal enzyme deficiencies (see table); *PEX1* analysis (common mutations c.2528G>A and c.2097_2098insT in Europeans); immunohistochemistry (anti-catalase, fibroblasts); complementation studies
Therapy: Symptomatic

Disorders of peroxisomal beta-oxidation

Clinical: Similar to disorders of peroxisome biogenesis
Enzymes: D-Bifunctional protein (*HSD17B4* gene), acyl-CoA oxidase (*ACOX* gene), sterol carrier protein x (one of two ketothiolases, *SCP2* gene, one patient)
Diagn.:   ↑ VLCFA; (↑) specific bile acids; normal plasmalogens

Rhizomelic chondrodysplasia punctata (RCDP)

Clinical features of RCDP are largely due to deficient etherphospholipid (plasmalogen) biosynthesis, catalysed by alkylglycerone-phosphate synthase (ADHAPS, imported via PTS2, *AGPS* gene) and glycerine-phosphate O-acyltransferase (DHAPAT, imported via PTS1, *GNPAT* gene). RCDP is usually caused by mutations in the *PEX7* gene coding for PTS2 (receptor of peroxisomal target signal 2); this condition is denoted RCDP1. RCDP2 (*GNPAT* mutations) and RCDP3 (*AGPS* mutations) are rare.

Clinical: Small stature (prenatal onset), proximal shortening of the limbs, facial dysmorphism, microcephaly, congenital cataracts, contractures, spasticity, mental disability, ichthyosis
Diagn.:   ↓ Plasmalogens; RCDP1: ↑ phytanic acid, ↓ pristanic acid (normal in single enzyme deficiencies); X-ray: stippling of the epiphyses; histology: irregular stippled calcifications of the dystrophic epiphyseal cartilage
Therapy: Phytanic acid restriction may be beneficial in some cases

Differential diagnosis of chondrodysplasia punctata (CDP)
- *CDPX1*: X-linked CDP in males, brachytelephalangic type, caused by arylsulphatase E deficiency (*ARSE* gene): hypoplasia of the distal phalanges without limb shortening or cataracts
- *CDPX2*: X-linked CDP in heterozygous females (lethal in males), caused by sterol Δ⁸-isomerase deficiency (see *page 119*)
- *Warfarin embryopathy* and other vit. K deficiencies (incl. vit. K epoxide reductase deficiency, deficient clotting, *GGCX* gene) may resemble CDPX1
- CDP tibia-metacarpal or humero-metacarpal type: short metacarpals, shortening of various long bones, no cataracts or skin changes; aut. dom., genes unknown
- *Maternal systemic lupus erythematosus* (SLE) and other maternal autoimmune diseases can cause CDP with rhizomelic limb shortening

X-linked adrenoleukodystrophy (ALD)

Most common peroxisomal disorder (incidence 1:20,000) X-chromosomal inheritance

Clinical: *Childhood cerebral form* (boys age 4–12): school failure, behavioural changes, visual/hearing impairment, intellectual regression, ataxia, adrenal insufficiency, leukodystrophy → decerebration within 2–4 yrs

Adrenomyeloneuropathy (AMN, males early adult, 20% of females, >35 yrs): progressive spastic paraparesis (legs), sphincter problems, impotence, mixed demyelinating and axonal peripheral neuropathy, adrenal insufficiency

Addison disease (childhood-adult, may be the only manifestation)

Bioch.: Deficient ALD protein = ATP-binding cassette transporter for import of VLCFAs (or their CoA compounds) into peroxisomes

Genetics: *ABCD1* gene (Xq28), de novo mutations in 7% of affected boys; no genotype-phenotype correlation, very variable within families

Diagn.: ↑ Hexacosanoic acid (C26:0, VLCFA plasma)

Therapy: Early haematopoietic stem cell (HSC) transplantation, HSC gene therapy; "Lorenzo's oil" (glyceryl trioleate + glyceryl trierucate 4:1) may reduce risk for childhood cerebral form when given to asymptomatic boys, may slow AMN progression in patients without cerebral involvement

Refsum disease

Clinical: Retinitis pigmentosa, polyneuropathy, cerebellar ataxia; deafness, anosmia, ichthyosis, skeletal and cardiac symptoms; normal intelligence

Manif.: School age

Enzyme: Phytanoyl-CoA hydroxylase (imported via PTS2, see above; *PHYH* gene)

Diagn.: ↑ Phytanic acid, ↓ pristanic acid; ↑ CSF protein concentration

Therapy: Phytanic acid-restricted diet; plasmapheresis

α-Methyl-acyl-CoA racemase deficiency

Clinical: Adult onset sensorimotor neuropathy, encephalopathy, neonatal hepatopathy

Pathogen.: Deficient 2R→2S isomerisation of pristanic acid and bile acid intermediates, required for β-oxidation; *AMACR* gene

Diagn.: ↑ Specific bile acids (bile, plasma, urine), ↑ pristanic acid, (↑) phytanic acid

Therapy: Substitution of bile acids

Other peroxisomal enzyme deficiencies

- Acatalasaemia (Catalase deficiency, *CAT* gene) → chronic mouth ulcers
- Primary hyperoxaluria type I (*AGXT* gene) → nephrolithiasis, nephrocalcinosis
- Mulibrey nanism (*TRIM37* gene): dysmorphic syndrome with growth retardation, pericardial constriction and abnormalities of muscle, liver, brain and eye

Protein glycosylation

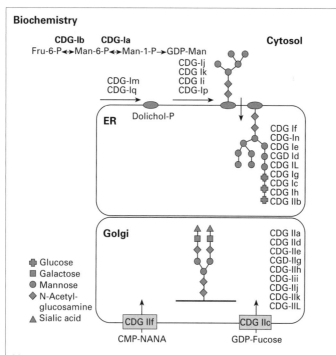

Biochemistry

Many enzymes, transport and membrane proteins, hormones, etc. require glycosylation to render them functional (glycoproteins). More than 100 enzymes are involved in the formation of carbohydrate side chains in the cytoplasma, endoplasmic reticulum (ER) or Golgi apparatus. Glycoprotein breakdown takes place in the lysosomes.

Fru = Fructose, Man = Mannose

Congenital disorders of glycosylation (CDG)

This group of disorders is characterised by *disturbance of various steps in glycoprotein biosynthesis that lead to a broad spectrum of symptoms*. The traditional classification was based on pathophysiological considerations: CDG type I represented defects in the assembly of the dolichol-linked glycan and its transfer to the protein in the cytosol or the endoplasmic reticulum whereas CDG type II referred to defects in the processing of the protein-bound glycans (mostly in the Golgi apparatus). The new classification is based on the combination of the approved gene name followed by CDG; e.g., PMM2-CDG is used for the previous CDG-Ia. So far, the molecular basis has been elucidated for 29 defects. By far the most common CDG type is PMM2-CDG (phosphomannomutase 2 deficiency).

Diagnosis
The diagnostic work-up should start with analysis of glycosylation patterns in *isoelectric focussing (IEF) of transferrin* (see *page 36*). The IEF patterns generally differ between CDG type I, (elevated disialotransferrin and asialotransferrin bands together with a decrease in tetrasialotransferrin) and CDG type II (trisialotransferrin and monosialo transferrin bands also elevated). Secondary glycosylation disorders may be caused by chronic alcoholism, classical galactosaemia or fructose intolerance (deficient mannose-6-phosphate synthesis).

Treatment
Treatment is symptomatic in most CDG types. Mannose administration is a successful therapy for PMI-CDG (Ib) and fucose has been used to improve the clinical picture of FUCT1-CDG (IIc) patients.

Phosphomannomutase deficiency (PMM2-CDG, CDG type Ia)

Most common CDG, ~80% of patients diagnosed so far. The disease may present in infancy with severe infections, liver/heart failure, bleeding tendency or thromboses; older children usually display non-progressive intellectual disability and neurological symptoms. The diagnosis is confirmed by enzyme studies (see table), treatment is symptomatic.

General:	Variable dysmorphism, inverted nipples, unusual fat pads, failure to thrive, diarrhoea, vomiting, thrombo-embolic events
Behaviour:	Often extroverted, happy character; stereotypic behaviour
Neurology:	Psychomotor retardation (IQ 40–60), hypotonia, deafness, epilepsy, cerebellar atrophy, ataxia, dysmyelinisation, haemorrhagic cerebral infarcts, neuropathy, ↓ nerve conduction velocity
Eye:	Strabismus, retinitis pigmentosa, cataracts
Heart:	Pericardial effusion, cardiomyopathy, heart malformation
Liver:	Hepatomegaly, fibrosis; histology: inclusion bodies
Kidney:	Proteinuria, nephrotic syndrome
Skeletal:	Kyphoscoliosis from school age, contractures, dysostosis multiplex, wheel-chair dependency
Endocrine:	Hypogonadism, absent puberty (females), hypoglycaemia
Haemostasis:	Abnormal coagulation studies, haemorrhages or embolic events
Clin. Chemistry:	↓ Various serum proteins (AT III, factor XI, protein C, protein S)

Legend to table (see page 148–150)
Shown are the main clinical features, the deficient enzyme and its cellular localisation, the IEF type pattern as well as the cell types used for enzymatic confirmation of the diagnosis.
Localisat. = localisation: C = cytosol; ER = endoplasmic reticulum; G = Golgi apparatus;
Confirm. = cells for confirmation of diagnosis: L = leukocytes; F = fibroblasts

Known CDG types

Enzyme	Gene	CDG type	Localisat.	Confirm.	Main clinical features
Phosphomannomutase	PMM2	Ia	C	L or F	Psychomotor retardation, dysmorphism, inverted nipples, cerebellar atrophy, coagulation abnormalities (see above)
Phosphomannose isomerase	PMI	Ib	C	L or F	Protein-losing enteropathy, hepatomegaly, congenital fibrosis of the liver; no psychomotor retardation; coagulation abnormalities, hyperinsulinism; therapy: mannose
α1,3-Glucosyl transferase	ALG6	Ic	ER	F	Hepatogastrointestinal symptoms, psychomotor retardation, strabism, coagulation abnormalities
α1,3-Mannosyl transferase	ALG3	Id	ER	F	Psychomotor retardation, hypsarrhythmia, postnatal microcephaly
Dolichol-P-mannose synthase I	DPM1	Ie	ER	F	Psychomotor retardation, seizures, axial hypotonia, dysmorphism, hepatosplenomegaly, coagulation abnormalities
Dolichol-P-mannose utilisation	MPDU1	If	ER	F	Psychomotor retardation, muscular hypotonia, hypertonia, contractures, seizures, skin disease
α1,6-Mannosyl transferase	ALG12	Ig	ER	F	Psychomotor retardation, hypotonia, dysmorphism, convulsions, feeding problems
α3-Glucosyl transferase	ALG8	Ih	ER	F	Gastrointestinal symptoms, hepatomegaly, coagulation abnormalities, severe diarrhoea
α1,3-Mannosyl transferase	ALG2	Ii	ER	F	Normal at birth, psychomotor retardation, ophthalmological abnormalities, seizures, hypomyelinisation, hepatomegaly, coagulation abnormalities

Enzyme	Gene	CDG type	Localisat.	Confirm.	Main clinical features
β1,4-Mannosyl transferase	*ALG1*	Ik	ER	F	Fetal hydrops, dysmorphism, large fontanel, psychomotor retardation, seizures, coagulation abnormalities, hypogonadism, cardiomyopathy
α1,2-Mannosyl transferase	*ALG9*	IL	ER	F	Normal at birth, developmental delay, severe microcephaly, central hypotonia, seizures, hepatomegaly, asthma
Dolichol kinase	*DOLK*	Im	C	F	Ichthyosis, cardiomyopathy, muscular hypotonia
RFT1-Protein	*RFT1*	In	ER	F	Developmental retardation, muscular hypotonia, seizures, hepatomegaly, coagulation abnormalities
Dolichol-P-mannose synthase III	*DPM3*	Io	ER	F	Muscular hypotonia, ataxia, cardiomyopathy, muscular dystrophy
α1,2-Mannosyl transferase	*ALG11*	Ip	ER	F	Muscular hypotonia, developmental retardation, seizures
Steroid 5α-reductase type 3	*SRD5A3*	Iq	C	F	Ichthyosis, cardiomyopathy, developmental retardation, cerebellar hypoplasia, coloboma
N-Acetylglucosaminyl transferase	*MGAT2*	IIa	G	F	Severe psychomotor retardation but no neuropathy or cerebellar hypoplasia; coagulation abnormalities, dysmorphism, seizures
Glucosidase I	*GCS1*	IIb	ER	F	Psychomotor retardation, hepatomegaly, hypoventilation, feeding problems, seizures, dysmorphism, normal IEF pattern
GDP-fucose transporter	*FUCT1*	IIc	G	F	Dysmorphism, psychomotor retardation, severe infections, normal IEF pattern; therapy: fucose (?)

Enzyme	Gene	CDG type	Localisat.	Confirm.	Main clinical features
β1,4-Galactosyl transferase	*B4GALT1*	IId	G	F	Macrocephaly, hydrocephalus, hypotonia, coagulation abnormalities, myopathy
COG complex in Golgi-trafficking, subunit 7	*COG7*	IIe	G	F	Dysmorphism, skeletal dysplasia, muscular hypotonia, hepatosplenomegaly, jaundice, epilepsy, death in infancy
CMP-Sialic acid transporter	*SLC35A1*	IIf	G	F	Macrothrombocytopenia, neutropenia, complete loss of Sialyl-LeX, bleedings of skin and posterior chamber, dyspnoea, infections
COG complex in Golgi-trafficking, subunit 1	*COG1*	IIg	G	F	Failure to thrive, developmental delay, muscular hypotonia, psychomotor retardation, progressive microcephaly, hepatosplenomegaly
COG complex in Golgi-trafficking, subunit 8	*COG8*	IIh	G	F	Failure to thrive, muscular hypotonia, mental and psychomotor retardation, progressive cerebellar atrophy, coagulation abnormalities
ATPase = subunit α_2 of H+-ATPase	*ATP6V0A2*	IIi	G	F	Cutis laxa, developmental retardation, seizures
COG complex in Golgi-trafficking, subunit 4	*COG4*	IIj	G	F	Mild hypertonia and hyperreflexia, respiratory disorders, mild ataxia, microcephaly, seizures
COG complex in Golgi-trafficking, subunit 5	*COG5*	IIk	G	F	Developmental retardation, intellectual disability, ataxia, hypotonia, cerebellar atrophy
COG complex in Golgi-trafficking, subunit 6	*COG6*	IIL	G	F	Recurrent vomiting, cholestasis, vit. K deficiency, intracranial bleeding, seizures

Neurotransmission

Monogenic disorders of neurotransmission have become recognised as a causes of severe early-onset progressive encephalopathies. The diagnosis is mostly based on the quantitative determination of the neurotransmitters or their metabolites in CSF incl. the amino acids glutamate, glycine and GABA and the metabolites of the biogenic amines and pterins. The clinical presentation of neurotransmitter disorders is quite distinct and they should not automatically be considered in every child with unexplained encephalopathy. Neurotransmitter analyses are not indicated in isolated intellectual disability or pervasive developmental disorders. Several disorders such as *GABA-transaminase deficiency*, *non-ketotic hyperglycinaemia*, or *pyridoxine/pyridoxal phosphate-responsive seizures* usually present with severe early-onset epileptic encephalopathy. Disorders of the biosynthesis of dopamine result in progressive extrapyramidal movement disorders. The spectrum of individual symptoms and disease courses is wide, ranging from intermittent focal dystonia to "hereditary spastic diplegia" and "cerebral palsy" to severe (lethal) infantile encephalopathies. For diagnostic guidelines see also *page 14*.

Disorders of biogenic amine metabolism

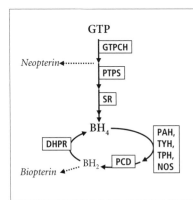

Biochemistry: Pterins

A disturbance of biogenic amine metabolism may be caused by a deficiency of tetrahydrobiopterin (BH_4), cofactor of the hydroxylation of tyrosine and tryptophan as well as phenylalanine (see also PKU; *page 67*) and nitric oxide synthase (NOS).

BH_4 is synthesised and regenerated by several enzymes. BH_2 = dihydrobiopterin.

For enzyme abbreviations see individual disorders.

Biochemistry: Biogenic amines

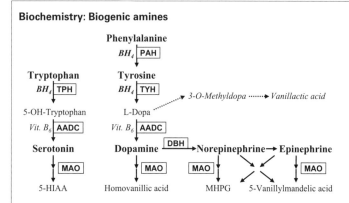

Aromatic L-amino acid decarboxylase is a vit. B_6-dependent enzyme and catalyses the formation of serotonin as well as dopamine; the latter may be converted by dopamine beta-hydroxylase into norepinephrine and epinephrine. For primary disorders of pyridoxine metabolism see *page 159*. The breakdown of biogenic amines involves monoamine oxidase-A and other enzymes. 5-HIAA = 5-hydroxyindoleacetic acid; MHPG = 3-methoxy-4-OH-phenylglycol. For enzyme abbreviations see individual disorders.

Clinical features
- *General:* progressive/severe epileptic encephalopathy, myoclonic epilepsy, psychomotor retardation
- *Dopamine deficiency:* parkinsonism-dystonia, dyskinesia and hypokinesia, dystonia and chorea, truncal hypotonia/limb hypertonia, may show typical deterioration during the day, oculogyric crises, miosis, ptosis, hypomimia, hypersalivation
- *Norepinephrine deficiency:* axial hypotonia, cerebellar symptoms, miosis, ptosis, ↓ blood pressure, hypoglycaemia
- *Serotonin deficiency:* insomnia, depression, disturbance of temperature regulation, disturbed intestinal motility

Dopa-responsive dystonia (Segawa disease)
Clinical: Dystonia starting in first decade (or later) (misdiagnosis "athetoid or dystonic cerebral palsy"); mostly pronounced diurnal variation
Enzyme: GTP cyclohydrolase (dominant mutations, incomplete penetrance)
Diagn.:   Quick remission on L-dopa; biogenic amines + pterins (CSF); normal Phe (consider Phe challenge; *page 47*), enzyme assay
Therapy: L-Dopa 4–12 mg/kg/day with a decarboxylase inhibitor (e.g. carbidopa); this usually achieves (almost) complete remission within weeks

Tetrahydrobiopterin (BH$_4$) deficiency ("atypical phenylketonuria")

Clinical: Features of dopamine and serotonin deficiencies
Enzymes: • GTP cyclohydrolase I (GTPCH, *GCH1* gene; recessive mutations)
                • 6-Pyruvoyl tetrahydropterin synthase (PTPS, *PTS* gene)
                • Quinoid dihydropteridine reductase (DHPR, *QDPR* gene)
                • Pterin carbinolamine dehydratase (PCD, *PCBD1* gene)
                • Sepiapterin reductase (SR, *SPR* gene)
Diagn.:   n–↑Phe (plasma; normal particularly in SR deficiency); biogenic amines (CSF), pter-
                ins (CSF, urine; see *page 14*); enzyme studies (DHPR in dried blood spot, all in fi-
                broblasts)
Therapy: • L-Dopa 8–12 mg/kg/day (neonates 1–3 mg/kg/day, infants 4–7 mg/kg/day), always
                with a decarboxylase inhibitor (e.g. carbidopa: 10–20% of L-dopa)
                • 5-OH-tryptophan (max. 6–9 mg/kg/day)
                • Tetrahydrobiopterin 5–10 mg/kg/day (monotherapy sufficient in mild PTPS and PCD
                deficiencies)
                • L-Dopa, 5-OH-tryptophan
                • Folinic acid 10–20 mg/day and Phe-restricted diet in DHPR deficiency (no BH$_4$)
                Caution: L-Dopa/carbidopa and 5-hydroxytryptophan should be introduced sequen-
                tially and increased slowly sometimes in steps of not more than 1 mg/kg over days/
                wks. 5-OH-tryptophan may not be tolerated due to gastro-intestinal side effects; mono-
                therapy with L-dopa/carbidopa may be sufficient in these cases.

Tyrosine hydroxylase (TYH) deficiency

Clinical: Severe dopamine deficiency with two phenotypes: a severe complex encephalopathy
                with onset in the neonatal period and an infantile onset, progressive, hypokinetic-rig-
                id syndrome with dystonia
Diagn.:   Biogenic amines (CSF); *TH* gene
Therapy: L-Dopa 1–10 mg/kg/day + carbidopa

Aromatic L-amino acid decarboxylase (AADC) deficiency

Clinical: Infantile onset, progressive, hypokinetic-rigid syndrome with dystonia, insomnia
Diagn.:   Biogenic amines (CSF); enzyme studies in plasma, *DDC* gene
Therapy: Bromocriptine, trihexyphenidyl, tranylcypromine, pergolide, vit. B$_6$, MAO inhibitors

Dopamine β-hydroxylase (DBH) deficiency

Clinical: Norepinephrine deficiency, especially severe orthostatic hypotension
Diagn.:   Biogenic amines (blood, urine, CSF); enzyme studies in plasma; *DBH* gene
Therapy: Dihydroxyphenylserine

Monoamine oxidase (MAO) deficiency

Clinical: Aggressive behaviour, mild developmental retardation, stereotypic hand movements,
                flushing (carcinoid syndrome)
Diagn.:   Biogenic amines (CSF and urine); whole blood serotonin, enzyme studies in fibro-
                blasts; *MAOA* gene
Therapy: Cyproheptadine hydrochloride, sertraline hydrochloride (risk of aggravating the sero-
                tonin/carcinoid syndrome)

Disorders of GABA metabolism

Biochemistry

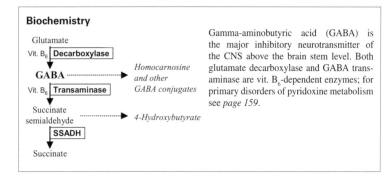

Gamma-aminobutyric acid (GABA) is the major inhibitory neurotransmitter of the CNS above the brain stem level. Both glutamate decarboxylase and GABA transaminase are vit. B$_6$-dependent enzymes; for primary disorders of pyridoxine metabolism see *page 159*.

GABA transaminase deficiency
Clinical: Neonatal fatal epileptic encephalopathy, psychomotor retardation, hypotonia, hyperreflexia, macrosomia, accelerated growth (↑ STH)
Diagn.:   AA (CSF): ↑ GABA; n–↑ homocarnosine, β-alanine; *ABAT* gene

Succinic semialdehyde dehydrogenase (SSADH) deficiency
Clinical: Variable: developmental retardation (mental, motor, language), hypotonia; seizures, hyporeflexia, ataxia, hyperkinesis, aggressive behaviour; sometimes autistic features, microcephaly/macrocephaly; MRI abnormalities (T2 hyperintensities in the globus pallidus and the white matter)
Diagn.:   OA (urine): ↑ 4-hydroxybutyric acid (excretion decreases with age; this may cause false negative results in semiquantitative analysis in older individuals); enzyme studies: fibroblasts, lymphocytes; *ALDH5A1* gene
Therapy: Symptomatic, incl. methylphenidate, thioridizine, risperidal and diazepines for problems of anxiety and behaviour
Progn.:   Slowly progressive encephalopathy, normal life expectancy

Other neurometabolic disorders

Glucose transport protein deficiency (GLUT1 deficiency)

Clinical: *Severe forms*: epileptic encephalopathy of infancy (70%) or early childhood (13%), (secondary) microcephaly, psychomotor retardation
            Milder variants: (exercise induced) movement disorders (ataxia, dystonia) without epilepsy (15%); childhood/juvenile/adult-onset absence epilepsy

Diagn.:   CSF analysis (following a 4–6 hrs fast): ↓ Glucose <2.7 mmol/l, glucose ratio CSF/blood <0.45 (normal 0.65 ± 0.1), n–↓ lactate/alanine. Glucose uptake test in erythrocytes. *SLC2A1* gene.

Therapy: Ketogenic diet; avoidance of drugs known to inhibit Glut1, e.g. barbiturates, ethanol, methylxanthines and tricyclic antidepressants

Progn.:   Satisfactory with early treatment

Hyperekplexia

Clinical: Exaggerated startle response, muscular hypertonia, generalised stiffness, normal EEG

Protein: α_1-Subunit of the glycine receptor (*GLRA1* gene, dominant or recessive), presynaptic glycine transporter 2 (*SLC6A5* gene, recessive), β-subunit of the glycine receptor (*GLRB* gene, recessive), and other proteins

Diagn.:   Mutation analysis; AA (CSF): ↓ GABA

Therapy: Clonazepam

Metabolism of vitamins and (non-protein) cofactors

Disorders of cobalamin absorption, transport and metabolism

Biochemistry

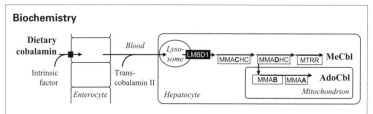

Dietary vit. B_{12} (cobalamin, Cbl) is bound to gastric intrinsic factor (IF), absorbed in the ileum via the cubam receptor, transported in the blood bound to transcobalamin II (TCII) and taken up by the cell through endocytosis. It is released from TCII in the lysosomes, transported into the cytosol, and converted to either methylcobalamin (MeCbl), cofactor of methionine synthase (see *page 70*) or mitochondrial adenosylcobalamin (AdoCbl, cofactor of methylmalonyl-CoA mutase; see *page 62*).

Disorders of absorption and transport of cobalamin
The most frequent cause of cobalamin deficiency in children is poor nutrition, e.g. prolonged breast-feeding of children when the mother herself is vit. B_{12}-deficient (for instance, because of a strict vegan diet).

Inherited disorders
(a) Intrinsic factor (IF) deficiency; *GIF* gene
(b) Imerslund-Gräsbeck syndrome: intestinal cbl malabsorption caused by deficient cubam receptor; components: cubilin (*CUBN* gene) and amnionless (*AMN* gene)
(c) Transcobalamin II (TCII) deficiency
(d) Transcobalamin I (TCI, haptocorrin, R binder) deficiency (glycoprotein that binds Cbl, released in stomach); unconfirmed disorder

Clinical: Vomiting, failure to thrive, psychomotor retardation, megaloblastic anaemia with hypocellular bone marrow, atrophic glossitis, progr. neuropathy/myelopathy/encephalopathy; sometimes hepatosplenomegaly; (b) usually proteinuria
Manifest.: Toddlers and pre-school children; c.) in the first months of life
Diagn.:   OA (urine): ↑ Methylmalonic acid; (↑) Hcy (plasma); ↓ TCII (c); ↓ cobalamin (normal in c); pathological Schilling test, corrected by IF (a)
Therapy: OH-Cbl (CN-Cbl) 1 mg/day i.m. for 2 wks; long-term therapy 1 mg/1–3 mths; in (a.): 1 mg once or twice weekly; folate up to 4 × 15 mg/day PO

Disorders of intracellular cobalamin metabolism (cbl defects)
cblF: Disorder of lysosomal cobalamin release; *LMBD1* gene
cblC: Most common disorder of cbl metabolism, deficient release of cob(I)alamine from cyano- or alkyl-cbl; *MMACHC* gene, prevalent mutation c.271dupA
cblD: Cytosolic protein; *MMADHC* gene, different mutations cause either combined AdoCbl and MeCbl deficiency or the respective isolated deficiencies

cblE: Deficient methionine synthase reductase, MeCbl synthesis; *MTRR* gene (see *page 70*)
cblG: Deficient methionine synthase, MeCbl synthesis; *MTR* gene (see *page 70*)
cblA: Disorders of mitochondrial AdoCbl synthesis; *MMAA* gene
cblB: Disorders of mitochondrial AdoCbl synthesis; *MMAB* gene

Clinical: (cblF, cblC, cblD) as in absorption/transport defects; (cblA, cblB) as in methylmalon-
              ic aciduria, see *page 62*; (cblE, cblG) failure to thrive, psychomotor retardation, hy-
              potonia/hypertonia, encephalopathy/neuropathy, epilepsy, megaloblastic anaemia; see
              methionine synthase *page 70*
Manifest.:   First months of life, sometimes neonatal
Diagn.:   OA (urine): ↑ methylmalonic acid (not in cblE, cblG, some cblD), ↑ homocysteine
              (plasma) (not in cblA, cblB, some cblD); cobalamin and TCII normal
Therapy: OH-Cbl i.m. 1 mg/day (CN-Cbl less effective); betaine (except cblA, cblB; see also *page
              70*); as in methylmalonic aciduria (cblA, cblB; see *page 62*); folate up to 4 × 10 mg/day PO

Disorders of folate metabolism and transport

Folate is predominantly found as 5-methyltetrahydrofolate (MTHF) in the blood and CSF. Human
folate transporters across membrane barriers include:
• Proton-coupled folate transporter (PCFT; *SLC46A1* gene), a high-capacity low-affinity system
  which mediates absorption of ditary folate at low pH in the upper small bowel but is also involved in active transport into the brain
• Reduced folate carrier (RFC; *SLC19A1* gene), bidirectional folate transporting system across
  membranes
• Folate-receptor 1 (alpha, *FOLR1* gene), a high affinity, low-capacity system, main transporter
  across the blood-brain barrier, endocytosis-based, also found in other organs (e.g. kidney)
• Folate receptor 2 (*FOLR2* gene), folate-binding protein in placenta, erythrocytes

Hereditary folate malabsorption (PCFT deficiency)
Clinical: Megaloblastic anaemia, failure to thrive, immunodeficiency, progressive intellectual
              disability, neurological disease
Diagn.:   ↓ Serum folate (normal: 5–15 µg/l), CSF folate (normal: 11–48 µg/l); hypersarco-
              sinaemia and ↑ formiminoglutamic acid (urine); *SLC46A1* gene
Therapy: Folate up to 4 × 10 mg/day PO; if inadequate CSF response, i.v. folinic acid 5 mg/day
              i.m. or 20 mg/kg PO qd

Cerebral folate transport (FOLR1) deficiency
Clinical: Early childhood onset, progressive movement disturbance, psychomotor decline, ep-
              ilepsy, hypomyelination
Diagn.:   ↓↓ CSF folate, serum folate normal, ↓ CSF BH$_4$; *FOLR1* gene
Therapy: Folinic acid 10–20 mg/kg PO qd

Dihydrofolate reductase deficiency
Clinical: Megaloblastic anaemia, pancytopenia, failure to thrive, immunodeficiency, progres-
              sive intellectual disability, epilepsy; cerebral and cerebellar atrophy
Diagn.:   ↓↓ CSF folate and BH$_4$; Hcy and serum folate normal; *DHFR* gene
Therapy: Folinic acid 10–20 mg/kg PO qd

Methylenetetrahydrofolate reductase (MTHFR deficiency)

Clinical: Infantile epileptic encephalopathy; progressive intellectual disability, variable progressive neurological and psychiatric presentations (especially posterior tract lesions), thromboembolism

Mild variant: see mild hyperhomocysteinaemia (*page 71*)

Diagn.: ↑ Hcy (>60 µmol/l); AA (plasma): n–↓ Met; nitroprusside test positive; *MTHFR* gene

DD: Folate malabsorption

Therapy: Betaine (up to 10 g/day in 3 doses); try riboflavin (vit. B$_2$) 5–10 mg/day, hydroxocobalamin (0.5–1 mg/day orally or 1 mg i.m. monthly) and folic acid 5–10 mg/day; folinic acid (15 mg/day) may be used instead but is more expensive.

Other disorders of folate metabolism

• *Formiminotransferase deficiency*: ↑ formiminoglutamic acid (urine); *FTCD* mutations, see histidine metabolism (*page 73*)

Other causes of reduced cerebral folate (5-MTHF) concentrations

• *Various non-genetic causes*: dietary folate insufficiency, intestinal resection, cancer, use of antifolate drugs, L-dopa, hepatic failure, coeliac disease
• *Autoantibodies to folate receptors*: onset in infancy: irritability, sleep disturbances; progressive intellectual disability, dyskinesia, cerebellar ataxia and spastic diplegia
• *Aromatic L-amino acid decarboxylase* (*AADC*) *deficiency* (see *page 153*)
• *Serine deficiency disorders* (see *page 74*)
• *Dihydropteridine reductase* (*DHPR*) *deficiency* (see *page 153*)
• Mitochondrial disorders

Disorders of biotin metabolism

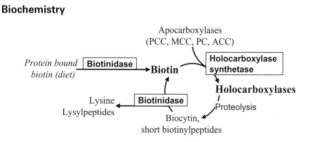

Biochemistry

The carboxylation of 3-methylcrotonyl-CoA, propionyl-CoA, acetyl-CoA and pyruvate is biotin-dependent. Multiple carboxylase deficiency may be caused by deficient activation of the apoenzymes (holocarboxylase synthetase deficiency, *HLCS* gene), deficient release of biotin from biocytin of protein-bound biotin (biotinidase deficiency, *BTD* gene) or by acquired biotin deficiency.

Multiple carboxylase deficiency (biotinidase, holocarboxylase synthetase)

Biotinidase deficiency is well treatable and measurement of the enzyme is included in the new-born screening programmes in many centres (enquire!). Holocarboxylase synthetase deficiency is only covered by tandem mass spectrometry newborn screening.

Clinical: Metabolic acidosis, progressive neurological symptoms, hypotonia, ataxia, seizures, intellectual disability, skin rashes, hair loss, immune deficiency

Manif.: *HLCS deficiency*: usually in the neonate
Biotinidase deficiency: usually in infants or toddlers, often insidious

Diagn.: ↑ Lactate, ↑ NH$_3$; AA (plasma): ↑ Ala; ↓ carnitine; OA (urine; CSF in rare cases): ↑ lactate, 3-OH-isovaleric acid, methylcrotonylglycine, methylcitric acid, etc.; enzyme studies: biotinidase (dried blood spot on filter paper card, plasma), carboxylases (fibroblasts, lymphocytes). Metabolic abnormalities may be fluctuating and inconsistent in biotinidase deficiency. *BTD* or *HLCS* genes.

DD: Defects of single carboxylases; secondary biotin deficiency associated with valproate therapy or as a result of gut sterilisation or the ingestion of massive amounts of raw egg-white

Therapy: *Biotinidase deficiency*: biotin 5–10 mg/day
HLCS deficiency: biotin 10–20(–40) mg/day

Disorders of pyridoxine metabolism

Biochemistry

Pyridoxine — PK → Pyridoxine-P — PNPO → Pyridoxal-P ← PNPO — Pyridoxamine-P
Pyridoxal — PK → ; Pyridoxamine — PK →
TNSALP / Cellular uptake / PK → **Intracellular pyridoxal-phosphate**

Pyridoxal phosphate (PLP; vit. B$_6$) is cofactor of >100 transamination and decarboxylation reactions in various pathways incl. serotonin and dopamine biosynthesis as well as alanine, serine, glycine and threonine metabolism. PLP is synthesised from dietary pyridoxal, pyridoxamine, or pyridoxine by pyridoxal kinase (PK) and pyridox(am)ine 5′-phosphate oxidase (PNPO); cellular uptake involves membrane-bound tissue non-specific alkaline phosphatase (TNSALP).

PNPO deficiency: Pyridoxal phosphate-responsive seizures

Clinical: Refractory neonatal seizures not responsive to pyridoxine but to pyridoxal phosphate;
              microcephaly, muscle hypotonia, prematurity

Diagn.:   Sustained cessation of seizures on pyridoxal phosphate
              AA (CSF): ↑ Ala, Thr, Gly; biogenic amines (CSF) mimicking AADC deficiency; OS
              (urine): ↑ vanillactic acid; gene: *PNPO*

Therapy: Pyridoxal phosphate 30 mg/kg/day oral in 3 doses (no pharmaceutical preparation
              available in Europe or the USA)

Hypophosphatasia

Clinical: Reduced skeletal/dental mineralisation:
              Prenatal: profound skeletal hypomineralisation, limb deformities, seizures, hypotonia,
              lethal in perinatal period
              Infantile: failure to thrive, rickets; seizures
              Childhood/adult: osteomalacia

Enzyme: TNSAP (*ALPL* gene); aut. rec.; some dominant mutations (late onset)

Diagn.:   ↓ Alkaline phosphatase (serum), ↑ phosphoethanolamine, PLP (serum, urine); X-ray:
              generalised undermineralisation, rachitic changes

Therapy: Pyridoxine in case of seizures

Antiquitin deficiency: Pyridoxine-(vit. B_6-)responsive seizures

There is no universal protocol for a pyridoxine challenge; high doses may be necessary at least
initially to control seizures. *Suggestion*: start with a single dose 100 mg i.v.; if patient is non-re-
sponsive, give additional 100 mg doses every 10 min up to 500 mg total. If there is uncertainty
about at least a partial response, pyridoxine 30 mg/kg/day should be continued for seven days before final conclusions are drawn.

Clinical: Epileptic encephalopathy presenting on day 1–2(–28); seizures respond only to pyri-
              doxine or pyridoxal phosphate
              Other features: jitteriness, hypothermia, neonatal dystonia, prodrome of restlessness,
              irritability and emesis preceding seizures; *atypical presentation*: neonatal onset but
              initial response to conventional anti-epileptic drugs; delayed response to treatment;
              late onset, i.e. later than 28 days

Enzyme: Antiquitin (*ALDH7A1* gene) = aminoadipic acid semialdehyde dehydrogenase in lysine
              metabolism (see *page 72*); deficiency causes accumulation of Δ^1-piperideine-6-car-
              boxylic acid (P6C), which inactivates PLP

Diagn.:   Sustained cessation of seizures on pyridoxine; ↑ aminoadipic acid semialdehyde,
              ↑ pipecolic acid (urine, plasma, CSF) (freeze samples immediately!)

Therapy: Maintenance: pyridoxine 5–10–15 mg/kg/day PO; folinic acid 3 mg/kg/day i.v. in 3
              doses, long-term oral medication maybe considered in cases with unsatisfactory re-
              sponse to therapy

Other causes of PLP deficiency

- *Hyperprolinaemia type II* (see *page 75*): accumulation of pyrroline-5-carboxylate (P5C) inac-
  tivates PLP; therapy: pyridoxine 10 mg/kg/day
- *Dietary deficiency* (rare), *decreased absorption* (coeliac disease), *isoniacid treatment, ginkgo
  fruit ingestion*: weakness, irritability, nervous disorder, insomnia, walking difficulty

Other disorders of vitamin metabolism

Disorders of thiamine (vitamin B₁) metabolism

Thiamine is required for acetylcholine synthesis and is a cofactor for the transketolation or decarboxylation of oxoacids (e.g. PDH and ODHC, *pages 97* and *98*; BCKDH, *page 66*; transketolase in the pentose phosphate pathway, *page 86*). Thiamine deficiency is not infrequent in children with metabolic disorders or other critical illness and is endemic in underdeveloped countries (beriberi).

Diagn.:   ↑ Lactate (blood, CSF), ↑ glyoxylate (blood, urine); ↓ transketolase activity (erythrocytes); clinical response to thiamine treatment

- *Thiamine-responsive megaloblastic anaemia*: anaemia, diabetes mellitus, hearing loss, onset mostly during infancy/childhood; thiamine transporter THTR1, *SLC19A2* gene; therapy: thiamine 25–75 mg/day
- *Biotin-responsive basal ganglia disease*: subacute encephalopathy, sometimes triggered by febrile illness; epilepsy, dystonia; MRI: basal ganglia lesions; thiamine transporter THTR2, *SLC19A2* gene; therapy: high dose biotin + thiamine
- *Amish type microcephaly*: severe congenital microcephaly, 2-ketoglutaric aciduria, fatal in infancy; *attenuated variant*: childhood onset, slowly progressive peripheral neuropathy, episodic encephalopathy, striatal necrosis; mitochondrial thiamine pyrophosphate carrier, *SLC25A19* gene

Familial isolated vitamin E deficiency

Clinical: Progressive neurological symptoms: weakness, ataxia, hyporeflexia, strabismus, loss of vision, cardiac arrhythmias, diabetes mellitus
Bioch: α-Tocopherol transfer protein (*TTPA* gene)
Diagn.:   ↓ Vit. E (plasma)
DD: Nutritive vit. deficiency, pancreatic failure, abetalipoproteinaemia
Therapy: High-dose vit. E (monitor plasma levels)

Miscellaneous disorders of vitamin metabolism

- *Molybdenum cofactor deficiency*: see sulphite oxidase deficiency (*page 71*)
- *Neurodegeneration with brain iron accumulation*: infancy onset progressive dystonia, dysarthria, spasticity, pigmentary retinopathy; attenuated adult forms. Deficient pantothenate kinase, required for CoA biosynthesis ("pantothenate kinase-associated neurodegeneration", *PKAN*); *PANK2* gene.
- *Vit. K epoxide reductase deficiency*: bleeding tendency caused by deficiency of all vit. K-dependent clotting factors; *VKORC1* gene (variants cause abnormal sensitivity/resistance to warfarin)
- Retinol binding protein deficiency: night blindness; *RBP4* gene

Metabolism of trace elements and metals

Disorders of copper metabolism

Wilson disease (hepatolenticular degeneration)

Clinical: Chronic liver disease, jaundice, cirrhosis; Kayser-Fleischer ring; dysarthria, poor co-
            ordination → bulbar paralysis; renal problems, haemolysis

Manif.:   6–18 yrs (liver disease), 20–40 yrs (neurological symptoms)

Enzyme: (Hepatic) Cu-binding P-type ATPase; *ATP7B* gene

Bioch.:   ↓ Biliary copper excretion, ↓ incorporation of copper into coeruloplasmin; accumu-
            lation of copper in liver, basal ganglia, kidneys

Diagn.:   Serum: (n–)↓ coeruloplasmin, n–↓ copper; ↑ copper (urine); liver biopsy (↑ copper);
            isotope studies (↓ incorporation into coeruloplasmin)

DD: An identical clinical presentation and similar therapeutic options have been described
            in two children with hypermanganesaemia (gene unknown).

Therapy: Avoid copper in food and drinking water (fish, liver); zinc, trientene; D-penicillamine
            (may cause hypersensitivity, bone marrow depression, autoimmune and connective
            tissue diseases); consider liver transplantation in severe liver damage

Monitor: Free copper = total copper – [coeruloplasmin x 3.15]; urine copper

Menkes disease

Clinical: *Classical form*: neonatal hypothermia, severe jaundice → progressive neurological de-
            terioration, epilepsy, peculiar facies, "kinky" hair, connective tissue/bone abnormali-
            ties → fatal (80–95%)

            Attenuated form: skin and hair abnormalities, ataxia, dysarthria

Var.:   • *Occipital horn syndrome*: laxity of skin and soft tissues, exostosis (occipital horn),
              diarrhoea, orthostatic hypotension; juvenile–adult onset
            • *ATP7A-related distal motor neuropathy*: minimal/no sensory symptoms; adult on-
              set, progressive

Enzyme: (Non-hepatic) copper ATPase, *ATP7A* gene, X-chromosomal! females usually asymp-
            tomatic (50% pili torti)

Bioch.:   Defective intestinal uptake of Cu → systemic copper deficiency, decreased synthesis
            of (~13) Cu-containing enzymes

Diagn.:   Serum: ↓ copper, coeruloplasmin (normal in adult neuropathy)

Therapy: Early copper-histidine subcutaneous injections (50–150 µg/kg/day)

Disorders of iron metabolism

The human body has no mechanism for removal of iron and thus needs to tightly control uptake. *Hereditary haemochromatosis* (*HH*) is characterised by accumulation of excess iron in parenchymal organs, resulting in serious illnesses incl. cirrhosis, hepatomas, diabetes, cardiomyopathy, arthritis and hypogonadotropic hypogonadism. Proteins involved in iron homoeostasis include (among others):

- *Ferroportin* (*SLC40A1* gene): exports iron from intestinal mucosa and macrophages
- *Hepcidin* (*HAMP* gene): main regulator of iron homoeostasis; secreted by the liver, binds and removes ferroportin and thereby reduces iron uptake from intestinal cells
- *Transferrin*: main iron transport protein in the blood
- *Ferritin*: main iron storage protein in liver
- *HFE* (*HFE* gene): regulator of cellular iron uptake via transferrin receptors
- *Transferrin receptor 2* (*TFR2* gene): mediates hepatic uptake of transferrin-bound iron, involved in the signalling pathway that triggers hepcidin transcription
- *Hemojuvelin* (HJV, *HFE2* gene): co-receptor in the signalling pathway that triggers hepcidin transcription

Hereditary haemochromatosis type 1

Clinical:	Hepatosplenomegaly, liver cirrhosis, hepatocellular carcinoma; arthropathy, cardiomyopathy, pituitary dysfunction (hypogonadism), diabetes mellitus, hyperpigmentation. Most common HH type (90%).
Manif.:	Age 40–50, male > female
Protein:	HFE = regulator of cellular iron uptake via transferrin receptor 1; *HFE* gene
Diagn.:	Serum: ↑–↑↑ ferritin, transferrin saturation, iron, transaminases
Genetics:	Common *HFE* variants p.C282Y (c.845G>A, allele frequency in Caucasians 4%), p.H63D (c.187C>G, allele frequency up to 25%), >20 rare mutations *Patients*: 80% homozygous p.C282Y, 5% comp. het. p.(C282Y)+(H63D) *Homozygotes p.C282Y*: symptoms only in 15–20% of males, 5% of females (biochemical evidence of iron overload in up to 50%)
Therapy:	If iron overload/symptoms: regular phlebotomy
DD:	*HH type 3*: like type 1, somewhat earlier onset/more severe, *TFR2* mutations *Acquired haemosiderosis*: e.g. in haemolytic anaemias requiring frequent transfusions, dietary excess in susceptible individuals (Bantu siderosis)

Juvenile haemochromatosis (HH type 2)

Clinical:	Severe iron overload in first to third decades; hypogonadotropic hypogonadism, progressive cardiomyopathy, arthropathy, liver fibrosis/cirrhosis. cardiomyopathy may predominate; abdominal pain in the first decade
Genetics:	90% *HFE2* (common mutation p.G320V), 10% *HAMP* (hepcidin)
Diagn.:	Serum: ↑↑ ferritin, transferrin saturation
Therapy:	Regular phlebotomy; deferoxamine in severe anaemia or cardiac failure

Hereditary haemochromatosis type 4

Clinical:	*Classical*: iron accumulation in macrophages of liver and spleen; liver fibrosis, mild microcytic anaemia
Genetics:	*Dominant inheritance*: *SLC11A3* mutations (loss/gain of function)
Diagn.:	Serum: ↑↑ ferritin, normal transferrin saturation (↑ in non-classical variant)
Therapy:	Regular phlebotomy; deferoxamine in severe anaemia or cardiac failure

Neonatal haemochromatosis (congenital alloimmune hepatitis)

Clinical: Hepatopathy of prenatal onset (IU growth restriction, oligohydramnios) neonatal liver failure; iron storage in various organs except reticulo-endothelial system; usually rapidly fatal; full recovery if survived

Diagn.:   Liver failure, relatively low transaminases, ↑ AFP, ↑ ferritin, ↓ transferrin

Pathogen.: Non-genetic: congenital alloimmune hepatitis (? maternal IgG antibodies)

Therapy: Unproven "antioxidant cocktail" + desferroxamine; liver transplantation

Advice: Recurrence in 60–80% of subsequent pregnancies, may be prevented with i.v. immunoglobulins

DD: Other causes of severe neonatal liver disease, e.g. mtDNA depletion (*page 106*)

Acoeruloplasminaemia

Clinical: Diabetes mellitus, retinal degeneration, extrapyramidal signs, dementia

Bioch.:   Deficient coeruloplasmin (ferroxidase $Fe^{2+} \rightarrow Fe^{3+}$), *CP* gene

Diagn.:   Serum: ↓↓ coeruloplasmin, ↓ copper, ↓ iron

Therapy: Phlebotomy, intravenous coeruloplasmin, desferroxamine

Disorders in the metabolism of other trace elements and metals

Disorders of magnesium metabolism

*   *Hypomagnesaemia*: cardiac and neurological symptoms; hypocalcaemia, hypokalaemia; mostly secondary (e.g. gastrointestinal and renal losses), rarely congenital disorders of renal tubular re-absorption of magnesium (classical Bartter's syndrome [*CLCNKB* mutations, presenting in infancy], Gitelman syndrome [*NCCT* mutations, presenting in childhood or adolescence])
*   *Hypermagnesaemia*: less frequent than hypomagnesaemia, results from failure of excretion or increased intake, can lead to hypotension, other cardiovascular effects, neuromuscular manifestations

Acrodermatitis enteropathica

Clinical: Typical skin rash, mucosal lesions, total alopecia, irritability, failure to thrive, diarrhoea, symptoms develop only after weaning

Bioch.:   ↓ Intestinal zinc absorption (uptake defect); *ZIP4* gene

Diagn.:   ↓ Zinc, (may be normal); ↓ alkaline phosphatase

Therapy: Zinc salts

Other trace elements

*   *Selenium* is a component of several glutathione peroxidases (see *page 77*) and type I 5'-iodothyronine deiodinase (converts T_4 to T_3). Clinical relevance of deficiency states is uncertain; may be a cause of (cardio)myopathies.
*   Manganese is a cofactor of prolidase (see *page 79*); deficiency state is not known.

Other metabolic pathways

LTC$_4$ synthase deficiency

Leukotrienes comprise a group of biologically highly active lipid mediators that are synthesised predominantly from arachidonic acid through the 5-lipoxygenase pathway. They include the cysteinyl leukotrienes (LTC$_4$, LTD$_4$, LTE$_4$) and LTB$_4$. Leukotriene synthesis may be affected by disorders of the gamma-glutamyl cycle (see *page 77*). Leukotriene analysis in CSF or other body fluids is not universally available.

Clinical: Progressive psychomotor retardation, hypotonia, no visual contact, failure to thrive, microcephaly

Diagn.:   ↓ LTC$_4$ (CSF), normal glutathione status, ↓ LTC$_4$-synthesis in nucleated cells

Sjögren-Larsson syndrome

Clinical: Spastic diplegia/tetraplegia, intellectual disability, epilepsy, photophobia, short stature; ichthyosiform keratoses (large skin folds, palmoplantar) from birth onwards

Enzyme: Fatty alcohol:NAD$^+$ oxidoreductase; *ALDH3A2* gene

Diagn.:   Enzyme activity (fibroblasts, leukocytes), ↑ leukotriene B$_4$ in urine

Trimethylaminuria (TMA-uria, fish odour syndrome)

Clinical: Unpleasant fish-like body odour due to volatile free trimethylamine (may increase with high choline diet, carnitine treatment, etc.); possibly deficient breakdown of biogenic amines and certain drugs; adrenergic reactions

Enzyme: Flavin-containing monooxygenase isoform 3

Genetics: *FMO3* gene, common variant allele [E158K, E308G] with reduced enzyme activity (allele frequency 20%) causes mild TMA-uria

Diagn.:   ↑ Free TMA (urine), ↓ ratio oxidised:free TMA (norm >90%)

Dimethylglycinuria

Clinical: One patient with body malodour as in trimethylaminuria, muscle fatigue

Enzyme: Dimethylglycine dehydrogenase, *DMGDH* gene

Diagn.:   ↑ CK; NMR spectroscopy (urine): ↑ dimethylglycine

Appendix

Helpful internet resources

Societies
- Society for the Study of Inborn Errors of Metabolism (www.ssiem.org)
- Society for Inherited Metabolic Disorders (www.simd.org)
- British Inherited Metabolic Disease Group (www.bimdg.org.uk) (emergency protocols!)

Disease-oriented databases and diagnostic laboratories

OMIM (www.ncbi.nlm.nih.gov/omim)
This is the online version of "Mendelian Inheritance in Man", the oldest and most widely used collation of genetic disorders.

GeneTests (www.genetests.org)
GeneReviews (www.ncbi.nlm.nih.gov/sites/GeneTests/review?)
GeneTests is a predominantly North American directory of clinics and laboratories that offer services and molecular tests for genetic disorders. It is linked to GeneReviews, a continuously expanding collection of excellent peer-reviewed articles describing clinical features, diagnosis, differential diagnosis, management, genetic counselling and molecular genetics of a large number of inherited disorders.

Orphanet (www.orpha.net)
Orphanet is a European counterpiece to GeneTests. The website is not as neat but it provides a wealth of information covering all aspects of rare disorders in various languages. It also includes a directory of DNA laboratories that offer molecular tests mostly in Europe. Another less comprehensive list of mostly European diagnostic laboratories is provided by EDDNAL (www.eddnal.com).

Genomic information and mutation data

National Center for Biotechnology Information (www.ncbi.nlm.nih.gov)
One of the main sources of molecular information on the internet.

Ensembl (www.ensembl.org)
This is a very useful genome database maintained by the EMBL and Sanger Institute.

Human Genome Variation Society (www.hgvs.org)
Human Gene Mutation Database, HGMD (www.hgmd.cf.ac.uk)
These websites provide links to various locus-specific databases that provide mutation data and other information on individual genes and disorders.

Free fatty acids and 3-hydroxybutyrate during fasting

Age-dependent normal values

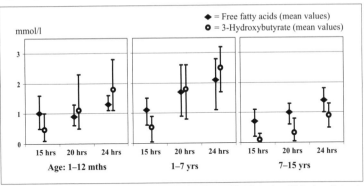

Shown are mean values and 10–90 percentiles for free fatty acids (plasma) and 3-hydroxybutyrate (deproteinised blood) in children after 15, 20 and 24 hrs fasting. Data from *Eur J Pediatr* 150 (1990) p. 80–5, with permission from Springer Verlag.

Correlation between free fatty acids and 3-hydroxybutyrate

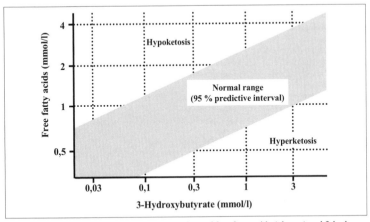

Shown is the correlation between the concentrations of free fatty acids (plasma) and 3-hydroxybutyrate (deproteinised blood) in children after a 24-hr fast. Adapted from *Arch Dis Child* 75 (1996) p. 115–9, with permission from BMJ Publishing Group.

168

Index

Special emergency medication

Special medication that may be used in metabolic centres

Drug	Preparation	Dose (emergency administration)
Betaine anhydrous	180 g powder for oral solution	250 mg/kg/day (oral; in 2 doses)
Carbamylglutamate	200 mg tablets	100 mg/kg/day (oral; in 3 doses)
Diazoxide		15 mg/kg/day (oral; in 3 doses)
L-Isoleucine		5–20 mg/kg/day (oral; in 3–5 doses)
L-Valine		5–20 mg/kg/day (oral; in 3–5 doses)
L-Methionine		100 mg/kg/day (oral; in 3 doses)
Nitisinone (NTBC)	2 mg capsules	1 mg/kg/day (oral; in 2–3 doses)
Riboflavin (vit. B_2)	e.g. 5 mg/ml or 14.6 mg/ml ampules (active ingredient)	150 mg/day (i.v.; in 3 doses) (e.g. 3 ampules three times daily)
Somatostatin	e.g. 3 mg powder	1–5 µg/kg/hr (i.v.)
Thiamine-HCl (vit. B_1)	e.g. 50 mg/ml ampules	Age 0–3 yrs: 150 mg/day; age >3 yrs: 300 mg/day; (i.v., in 3 doses)